# VOLUME 1

## Dr. Lana
## Weight Loss
## Workbook

Day 1 - 90

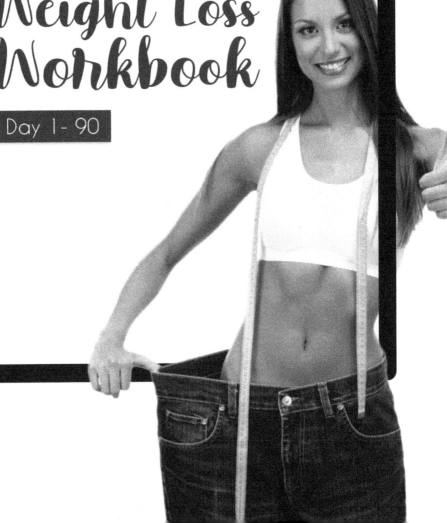

# INTRODUCTION

## VOLUME 1

My name is Lana Moshkovich and I am a Doctor of Acupuncture and Chinese Medicine. I practice in the state of IL in a beautiful Clinic in Deerfield.

All my life I struggled with weight loss and finally created a wonderful support system for myself. I lost 34 lbs in 7 months.

I would like to share it with you. This book is not the same as others' books. Instead of writing a general weight loss book I thought to share with you my personal daily, weekly, monthly routines.
Lana's Weight Loss Guide and Workbook is a series of 3 month volumes.

It's organized and developed in a daily format with motivational help, my daily food intake and recipes, pictures and gym routines.

Anyone can replicate the work I have done and it's doable.

# INSTRUCTIONS

My e-Book is easy to use.

Every day you will see my story and my routines for the day and you have an opportunity to write down what you are going to do and what you have done.

You can enter your metrics every day (weight, BMI, size...)

Morning Brainstorm. On your workbook page you have Morning Brainstorm where you get ready for this particular day. This is your planning thoughts

Evening Reflection. Here you will have an opportunity to write what you have done for your weight loss , meals that you eat, workout you have done.

# DAY 1-90

Use this book twice a day in the morning and in the evening to write down your daily routine.

At the end of each month you will see my summary with video for my accomplished results. You also have a page for your own summary progress for your entire month.

# COMPLETION AND CONGRATULATIONS

You have finished 3 months of my weight loss program. Join me in my next e-guide and workbook for 3 more months.

Page for someone

# TODAY I FEEL

Gloomy
Tired
Ok
Great
Ready to rock

What can I do to feel ready to rock?

Morning brainstorm

Evening reflection

# DAY 1

# Manifesto

I decided to lose weight and actually commit to it. I created a motivational group for people in our community who are trying to lose weight and keep it off.

I created this group to get started on my weight loss journey and to inspire anyone who wants to share their success and be motivated, positive and trying to reach their weight loss goal.

Let's motivate and help each other to get in better shape.
community who are trying to lose weight and keep it off.

Let's help each other to feel strong, happy and accountable for our choices.

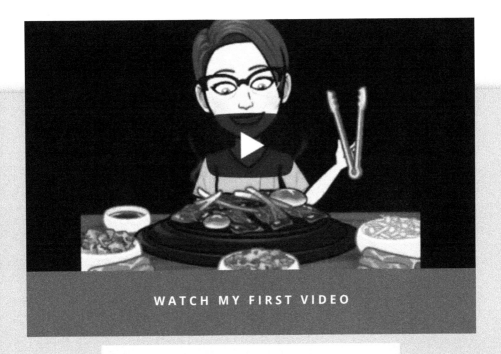

**WATCH MY FIRST VIDEO**

https://youtu.be/gndCthN8SlY

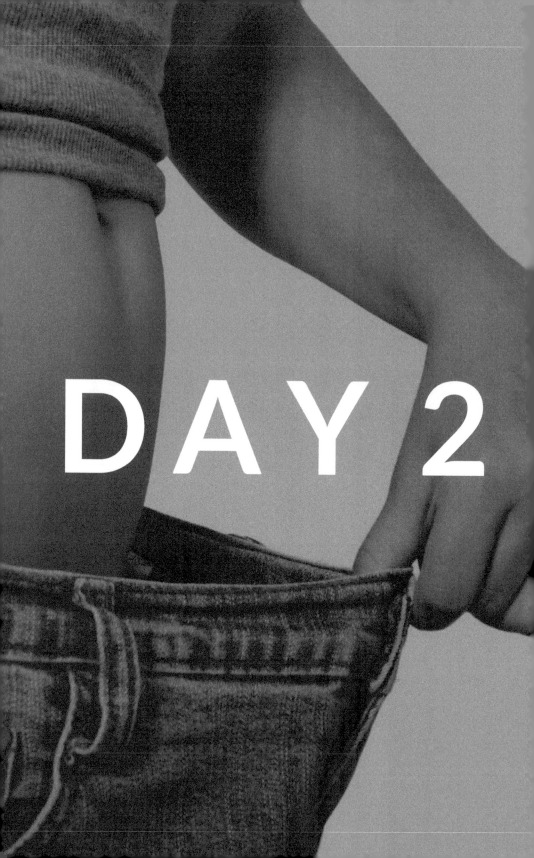

Your weight loss success starts with the kitchen. I started with cleaning my shelves. I organized everything and threw away not healthy items. I did grocery shopping. Now it's easier to eat healthy, be happy and lose weight.

It's important to stay POSITIVE!

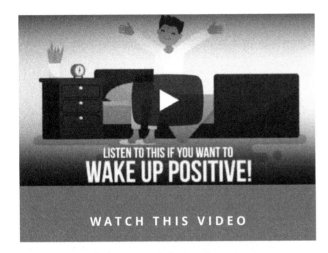

**https://youtu.be/AVRYrrrQeds**

Clean kitchen. Almost nothing on the counter. I am so ready.

It's a World Food Day!
Let's remember to eat healthy!
Colorful meals are the best!

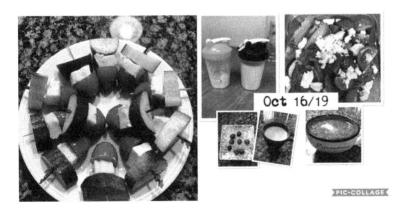

Make sure you celebrate it with kids.

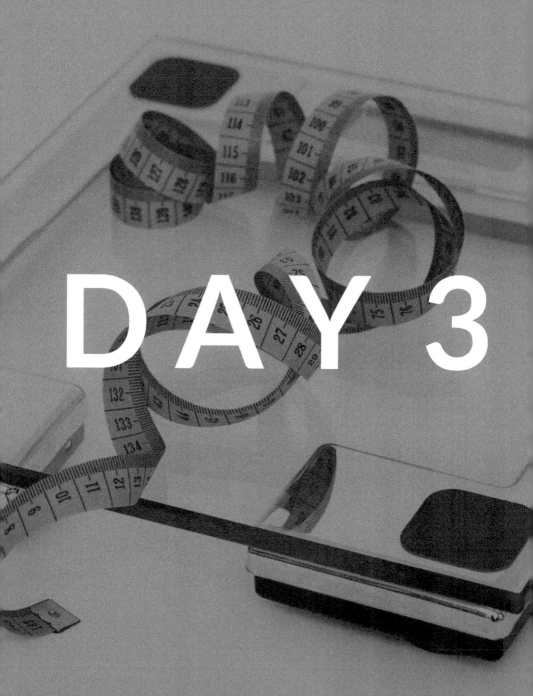

Today I suggest listening to this great episode in your car while driving to work or later when going home!

It's great to see what people can accomplish.

🤍 There are a lot of kids who fall into the wrong path. I encourage you to send it to parents with problems in their family. I sent a text to my patient today with a link to this video. She was so happy when she received it. Now she will put it on when she drives her teen somewhere. 🤍

I believe there is nothing impossible if you believe, want and do everything you can for anything that you want to happen.

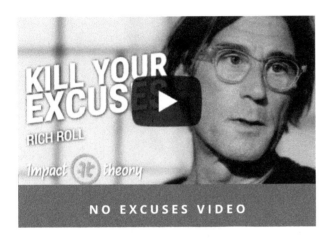

https://youtu.be/k7iq2Z2D1Zs

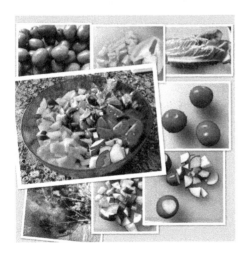

Find and join my 👉 Lana's Weight Loss Happy Club 🤚 where I post daily. I hope to inspire people to lose weight.

There are no sales or anything specific to any particular diet. Pure motivational support and positivity in the group.

I learn to meet positive people and inspiring is the key to success in any direction.

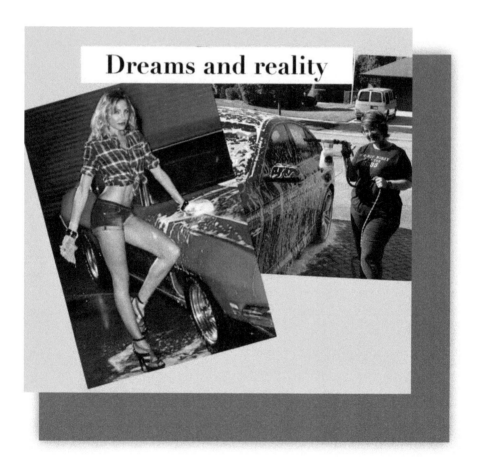

# DAY 5

😄 Great thing to start during fall season. I am almost done! 🙌

😷 The main idea is to clean your fridge and pantry from distractions.

It's good to develop and start a 30 day Declutter challenge.

Day 1 Clean out your bathroom cabinets

Day 2 Purge your closet or clothing you don't need

Day 3 Clean out shower

Day 4 Clean out TV cabinets

Day 5 Clean off kitchen table

Day 6 Clean out your wallet

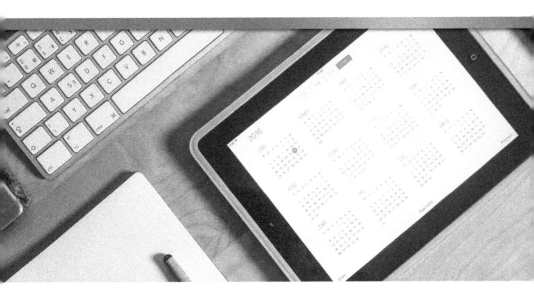

## CREATE YOUR OWN 30 DAY DECLUTTER CHALLENGE:

Day 1. _____
Day 2. _____
Day 3. _____
Day 4. _____
Day 5. _____
Day 6. _____
Day 7. _____
Day 8. _____
Day 9. _____
Day 10. _____
Day 11. _____
Day 12. _____
Day 13. _____
Day 14. _____
Day 15. _____
Day 16. _____
Day 17. _____
Day 18. _____
Day 19. _____
Day 20. _____
Day 21. _____
Day 22. _____
Day 23. _____
Day 24. _____
Day 25. _____
Day 26. _____
Day 27. _____
Day 28. _____
Day 29. _____
Day 30. _____

Do you think that you are functioning at your fullest potential? 🫤

🍪 Beautiful salad in a glass. Makes it more appealing even though salad can be great no matter what the presentation is.

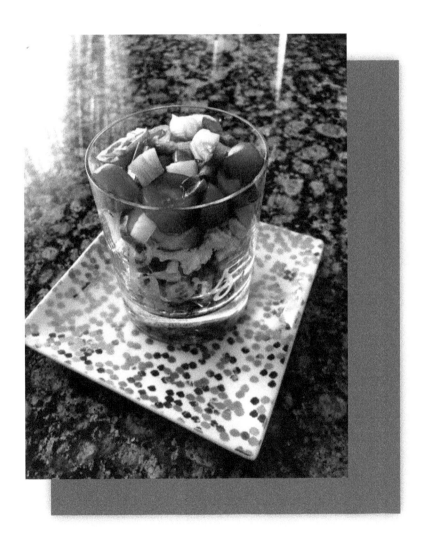

DAY 7

👩 Good Morning and happy Monday!

Get your head together!

Why is Weight Loss all in your Head?

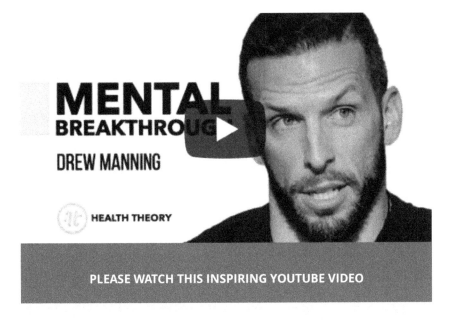

**PLEASE WATCH THIS INSPIRING YOUTUBE VIDEO**

**https://youtu.be/cqwQosiUhTk**

👉 Today I decided to create my vision board. I found a few pages from a Shape magazine and placed them there.

🩶 I have a picture of this super good looking woman lifting a bar. I would be thrilled if I ever do anything like that.

I have my wall calendar there.

I would need some stickers for fun.

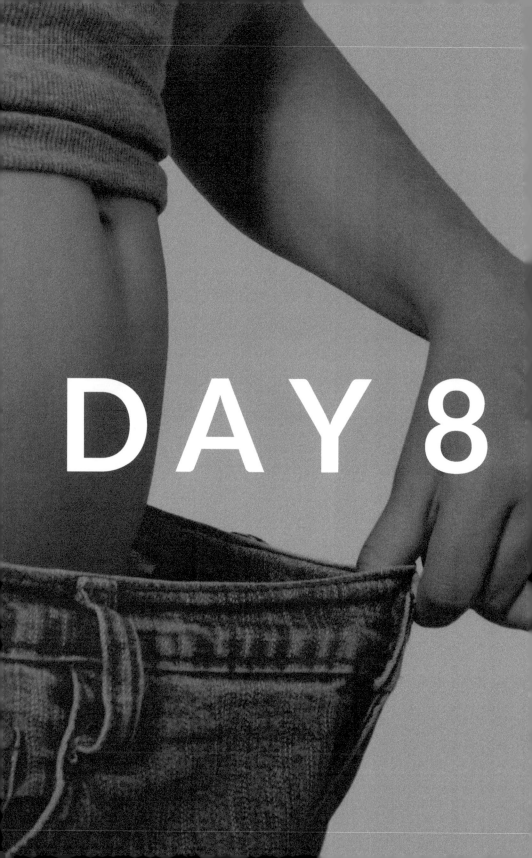

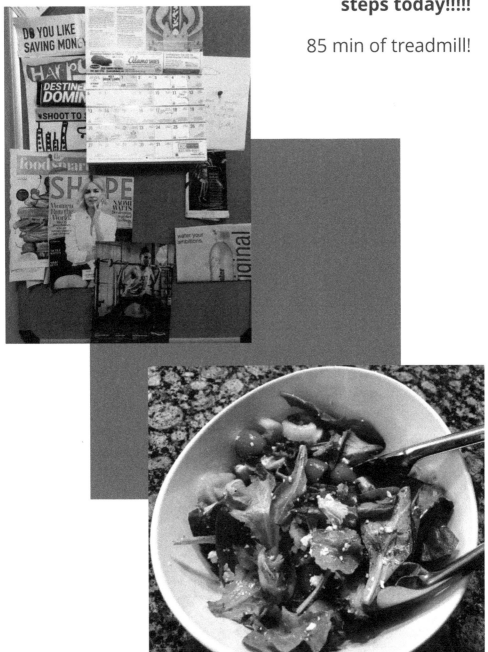

**Well done with 15500 steps today!!!!!**

85 min of treadmill!

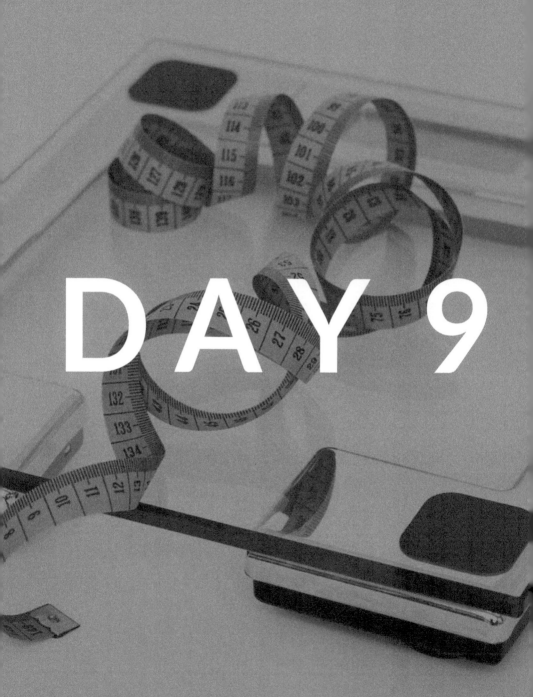

DAY 9

🤍 Happy Wednesday!

👉 I am so proud of myself for walking 85 min on the treadmill  yesterday at a very late time.

👉 Prepped my lunch for today at 11 pm yesterday

👉 Cooked dinner for everyone

Usually Wednesday is my morning shift at work but today working 9-7:30 so will not have a chance

I am feeling fantastic! Hope you are too!

Here is a great video to watch or listen while getting ready to work!

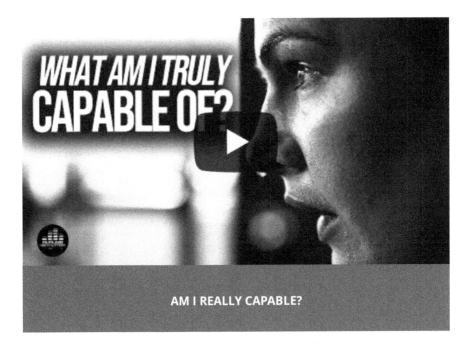

**AM I REALLY CAPABLE?**

**https://youtu.be/Bet7pl3p4_g**

DAY 10

# Why don't people get results?

1. They are only doing cardio

2. Lack training consistency

3. Having no structural program

4. Always giving up too soon

5. Not making this a lifestyle

6. Eating too many calories

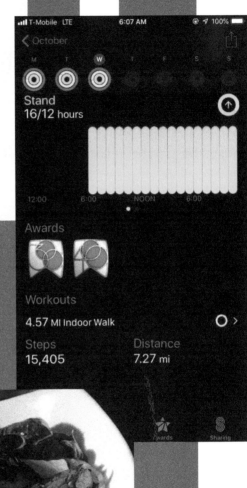

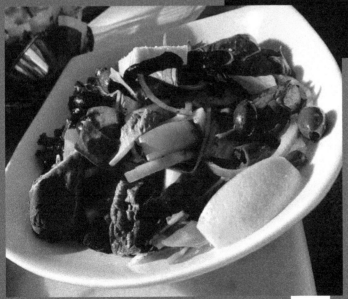

I took 10 min to brainstorm my meal plan for today and decided on these simple breakfast, lunch and dinner.

I have vegetables, hummus, feta and some liver pate

Planning, planning, planning my day.

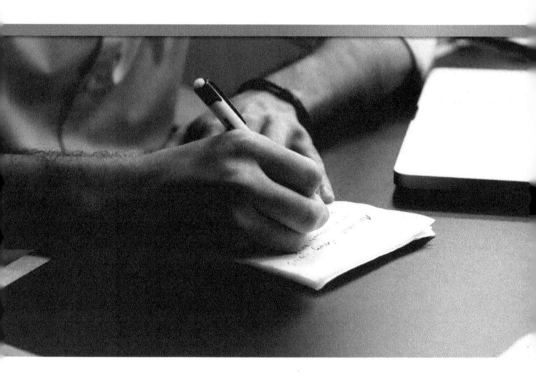

# DAY 12

Coffee for breakfast.
Lunch- mushrooms and sour cabbage salad.
Dinner -½ cup of  buckwheat and liver pate/

I walked outside for 30 minutes. Walking is so beneficial.

I believe we cannot lose a lot of weight from walking unless walking is a huge struggle. In my opinion walking improves mood and motivates more, keeps accountability.

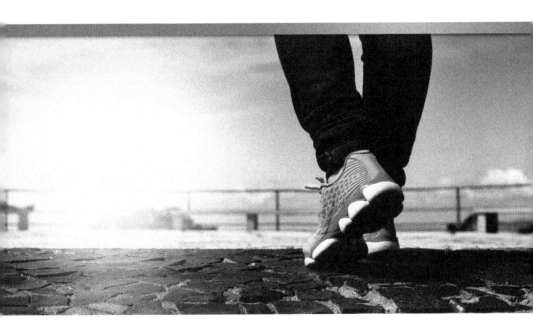

Some of the Healthy Tips and Habits I will follow:

Portion Control
Great attitude
Promise and deliver
Walk is a form of physical activity
Complex carbs in moderation
Simple carbs on occasion
Keep journaling
Surround myself with positive supportive people

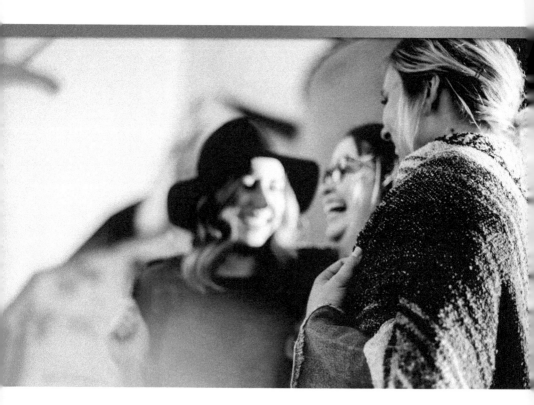

DAY 14

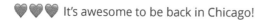 It's awesome to be back in Chicago!

Happy to find out that I didn't ruin my weight loss while being in NY and eating out 3 days a week.

I had to sit A LOT!!!!!!

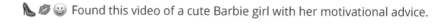 Found this video of a cute Barbie girl with her motivational advice.

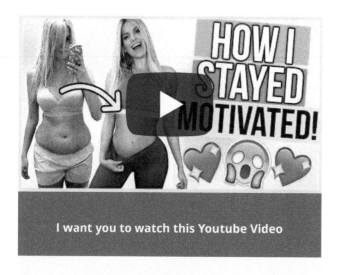

**I want you to watch this Youtube Video**

**https://youtu.be/SvE_xFkxfJA**

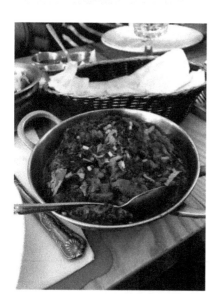

For those who are still thinking they want to lose weight:

I have been on the different diet plans my whole entire life.

I was very successful when I was 25 year old and had 2 years old ( if I am not mistaken)
In 6 months I lost about 60 or 65 lbs.

In my opinion, the most important key to success is not a specific diet but a specific mindset or serious desire to achieve.

You have to be ready!

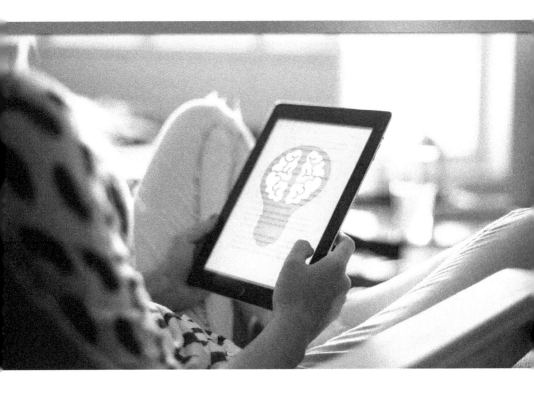

I suggest finding motivational videos on YouTube and listening to them every morning.

It is boosting your confidence and being more exciting.

I also learn it's important to follow specific people. There is a lot of information on diets or advice.

Find people who have lost unwanted weight and kept it off.

Meditation and praying will not help you lose weight.

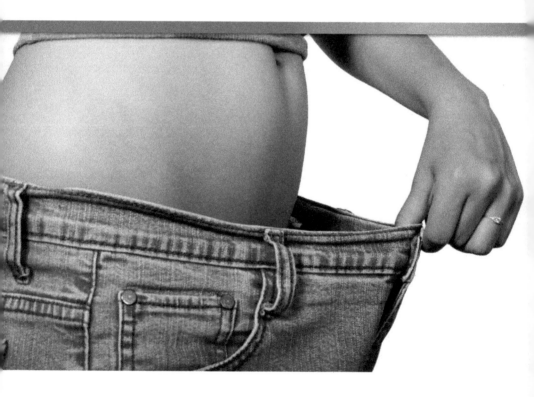

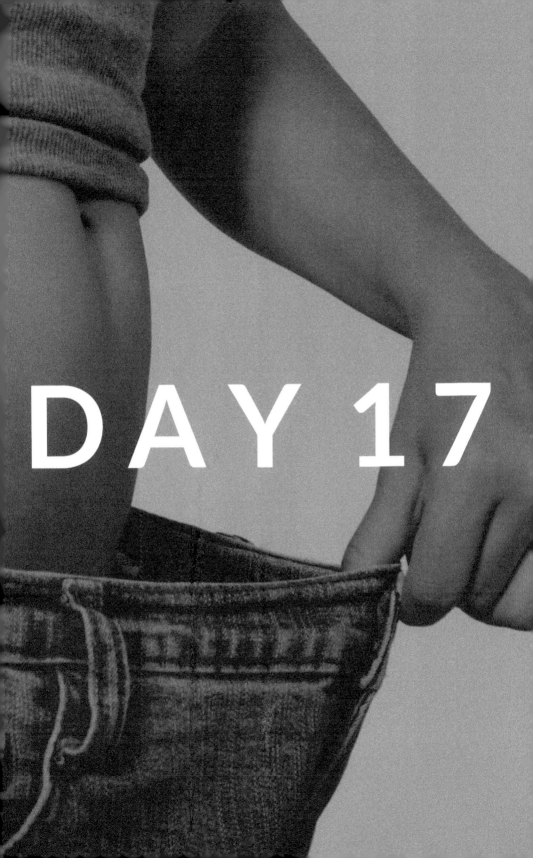

😊 Happy Halloween everyone.

This is me probably 4 years ago or so. I want to reach my goal.

Post your Halloween 👻 picture of what you want to be. I am sure you have one best looking crazy picture. If not it's ok. 🧟

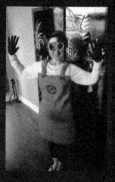 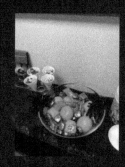 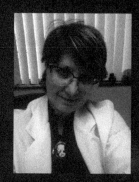

I hope we find a way to walk more today even though we have first ❄️.

Have a good work day, everyone. Stay out of candies. Or taste the best one- Dark chocolate!

Halloween 🎃 can be a healthier version. We tried.

I am not touching any candies.

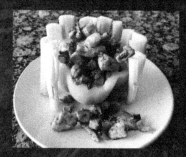

Halloween 🎃 dinner!

Treadmill 45 min!

No candies or even fruit!

Staying 💪 strong!

Snack: 2 mandarins.

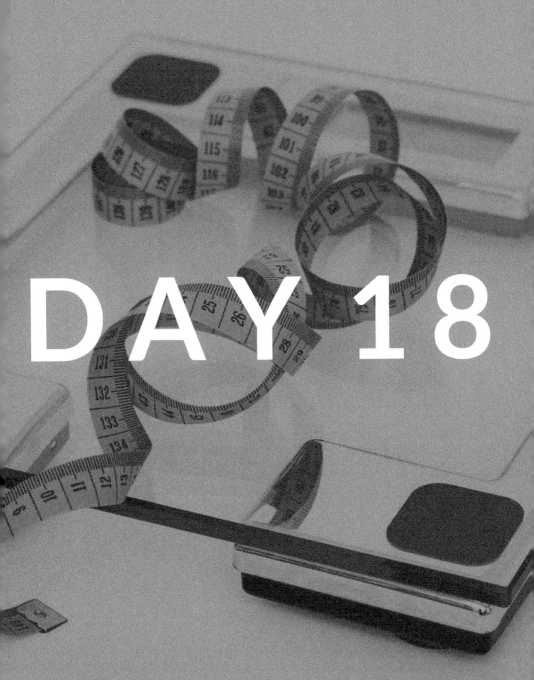

DAY 18

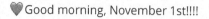🩶Good morning, November 1st!!!!

Cold but beautiful outside! ❄️

Thanks to my IWatch for monthly challenges.

October challenge Won!🏆 16 workouts in a month. Not to mention I started Oct 15.👏

Get your dose of vit D and let's work on Friday like champions. For many of you this is the last day of work week. For me and others who work on Saturday: We can do it! What can be better than beautiful day of work!🥴

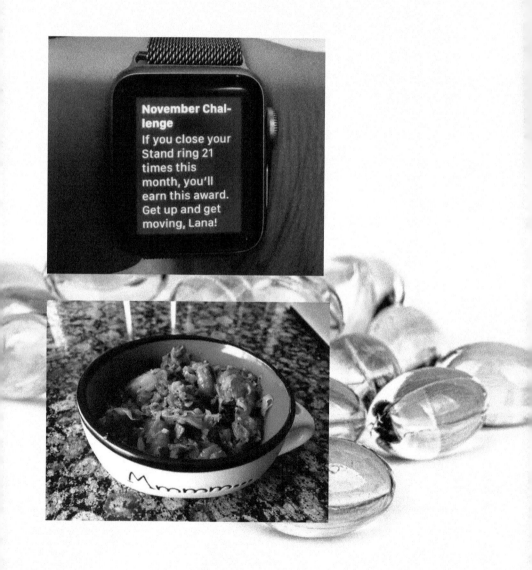

# DAY 19

😃 Happy Saturday, everyone!!!!

😓 Some of you are off today.

🧘 Let's eat healthy and be happy. Nutrition is the most important for weight loss. Working out is always secondary. But don't skip it!

Set up your plan. Dream big.

November is new month, new beginning, new mindset, new focus, new start

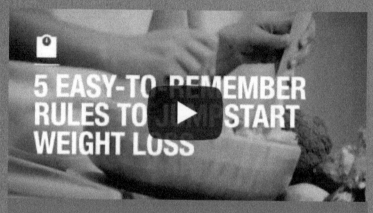

**Watch these 5 easy steps to jump start weight loss**

**https://youtu.be/60SBjfp2WRE**

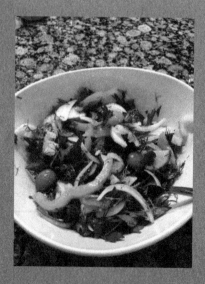 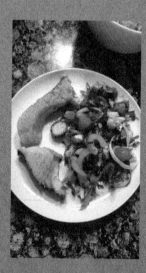

DAY 20

Good Morning Everyone!!!!

😀 I love Sundays!

58 Days before New Year 2020 Celebration! 🪄🎉🎅 Are you ready to lose unwanted 5, 10 or 20 lb?

Look at Santa. He dropped tons of weight. Looking HOT!

Anything is possible if YOU BELIEVE!

🎅 I would love to create a friendly competition with a prize. Everyone will benefit from this because we are all going to WIN!

---

## 1ST CHOICE

🏆 I propose % of your weight loss 🏆

We can get together for a great celebration at the end of competition( in January) and have FUN. 🥴

😖 The best part of it: NOBODY needs to know your weight. It's all on you. YOU are in charge of your weight and your percentage.

Give me an idea of an app or something that might show percentage of your weight loss.

---

## 2ND CHOICE

🏆 Workouts time during 58 days.

Your app will show that

---

## 3RD CHOICE

🏆 Steps during 58 days

Your apps will do that too.

👉 🤍 Comment please on choices of preferred competition game rules.

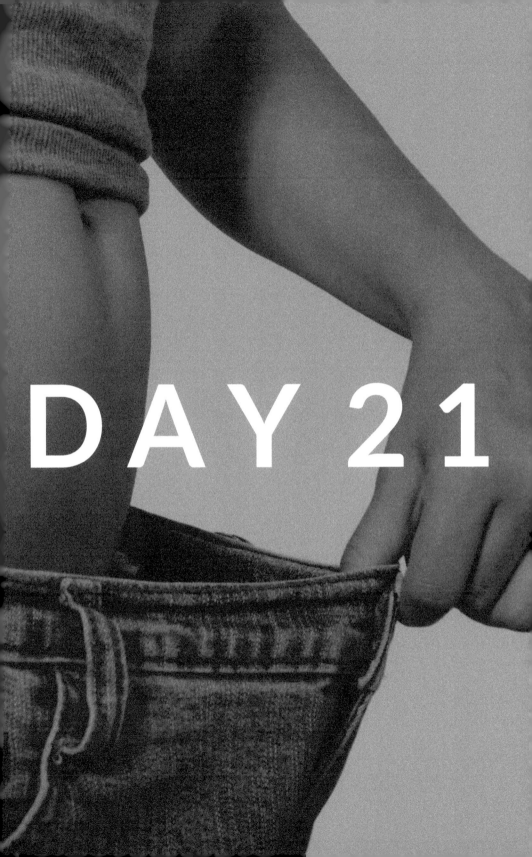

All people want to have a healthy weight for different reasons.

I am definitely on a path of LOOKING AMAZING!!!

Share your dreams if you want. 😌

I learned a great lesson yesterday. Going to a 🎂 birthday party is a great weight loss starter!

Great friends, conversations, happiness and healthy food choices are more important then overeating! 🎂

I skipped the wine and handmade tiramisu 🍰.

And felt great. Didn't workout yesterday due to Don't want to ruin my new hair day and lose weight.

My point is

1. Food choices are more important than exercise

2. Invite me for a 🎉 party😄

3. Believe in yourself

What motivates you the most?

1. Feeling confident?I want to look and feel the best

2. Looking Amazing? I want to look amazing at the event.

3. Getting revenge? I want my ex to regret losing me.

4. Improving health? I want to prevent health issues.

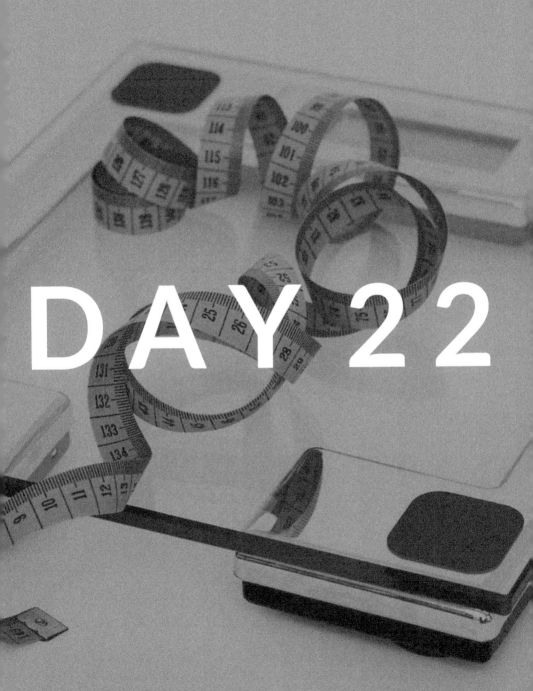

DAY 22

Happy Tuesday, friends!

🍩 🍫 🍪 Sometimes we crave things we better don't eat.

Please share things that helped you during those times.

👉 Coffee works for me and busy work schedule

👉 Glass of water or cup of tea with stevia

👉 Boiled egg

---

Step by step

Expect falling down and then rising up

Because we are worriers!

Who loves those?

I found it in my home gym without any use. I remember a time when I could do 200 spins.

Time to start using it.

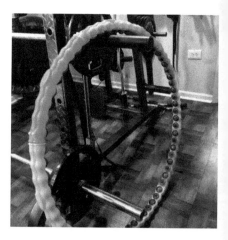

DAY 23

🔑 Consider learning from people who are the best in what you want to accomplish.

😄 Hope you find someone who does know how to lose weight!

😜 There are plenty of MDs, Nutritionists, Dietitians, and/or personal trainers who claim to know what to do.

Everyone in this group KNOWS EXACTLY what to do.

🤪 Knowing and doing are two different things🤪

Let's just do it 🤍

👉 Breakfast. Coffee

👉 Lunch at work. Salad with cucumbers, radishes, parsley and tuna

👉 Dinner. Cabbage Salad and cauliflower

👉 Walking with friends is also awesome!!!

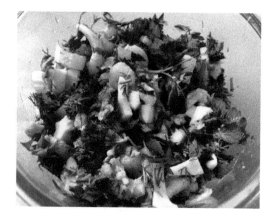

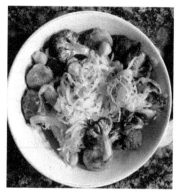

DAY 24

Great video to listen while driving to work or during a workout:

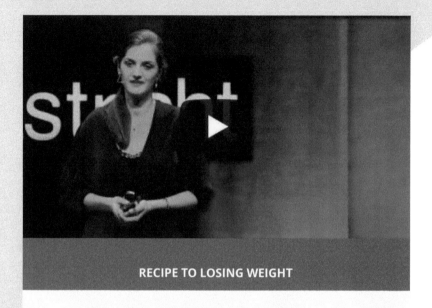

**RECIPE TO LOSING WEIGHT**

**https://youtu.be/KfK3eK-kOQA**

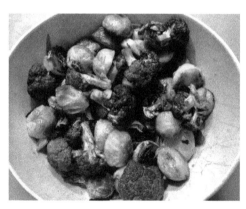 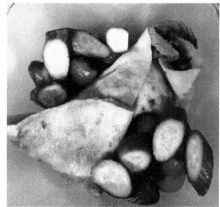

DAY 25

Nothing excites me more than someone's true weight loss story.

👉 Trying intermittent fasting for 16 hours

It's definitely not a big problem except creamer in my morning coffee ☕

Wishing you a good day!

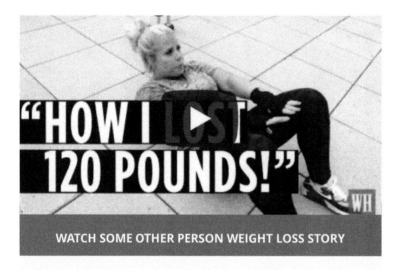

WATCH SOME OTHER PERSON WEIGHT LOSS STORY

**https://youtu.be/r9jerUKJDuI**

Just a joke:

My new diet plan: Make cupcakes for all my friends; the fatter they get, the thinner I look!

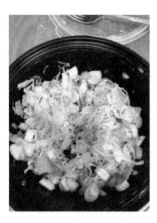

NO PILLS- NO EXERCISE

IN ONLY ONE MONTH YOU CAN DO IT TOO!

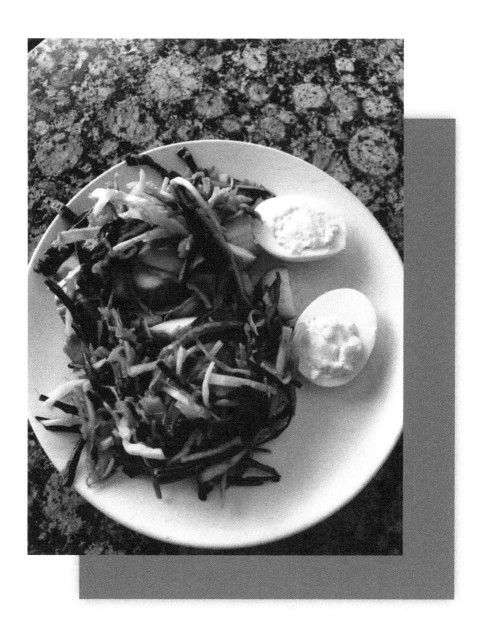

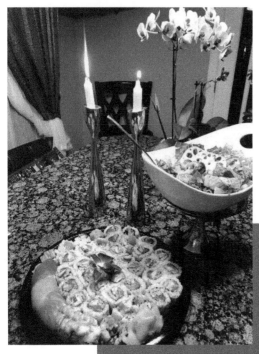

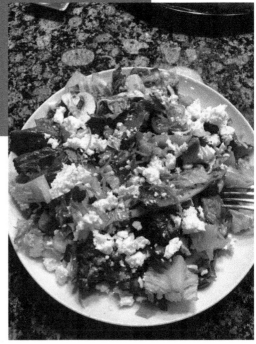

https://www.higherperspectives.com/walking-daily-2626517339.html?
fbclid=IwAR2omY-Iwo2tiNKKU30XjhyAdvPFeC7j1Bbba1l3G5djoKO8PpOxsr94hfI

🚶, I have been walking on treadmill daily since October 15. Minimum 45 min- Maximum 1 hr 25 min depending on the show length I watch.

🩶 I feel so much better.

Hope you are too. Many of you started walking more too which made me feel good. I hope my posts have a little impact on your desire to be better everyday.

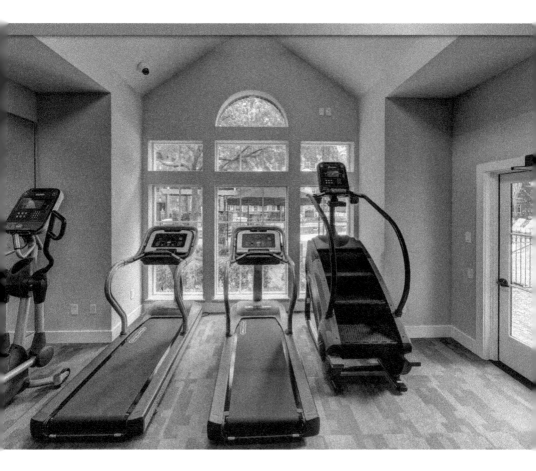

🙏 God, please help me today! 🙏

I have a feeling that I overate today.

- 2 protein shakes
- chicken soup 🍲 for lunch
- chicken 🍗 and salad 🥗 for dinner

I feel so full. I hope 🤞 it's enough to not gain any weight.

👇😅🤑 Look at this lovely board someone created for weight loss visual.

💚 Good evening!

I had an absolutely wonderful day!

👍 I tried and accomplished 16 hours of fasting!

👍 Tried new workout on stationary bicycle 🚲

👍 Eating very healthy but not limiting myself to any food. I had my homemade soup with a cup of broccoli.

👍 Best accomplishment ever- my diabetic patient is walking more now and got 7000 steps yesterday!

👍 I hope people receive good motivation from me or any member of this group.

## DON'T FORGET, YOU ARE WHAT YOU EAT

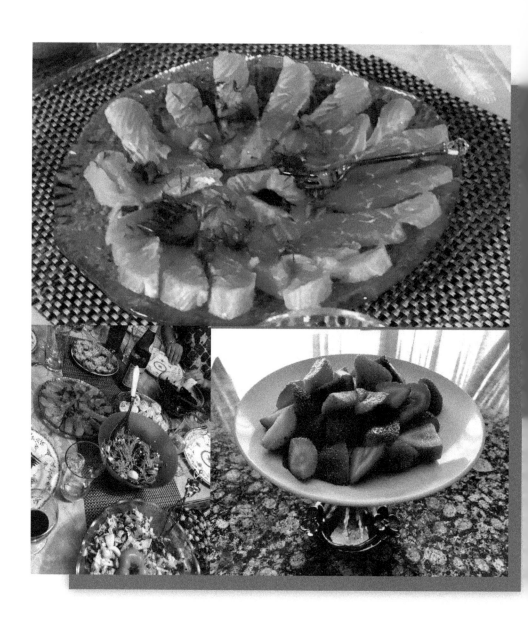

🪨 Today is my 1 month anniversary of a dedicated weight loss journey!

I am a proud loser of 12.5 lb 🤞 😄 👏

😎 Thank you for being supportive!

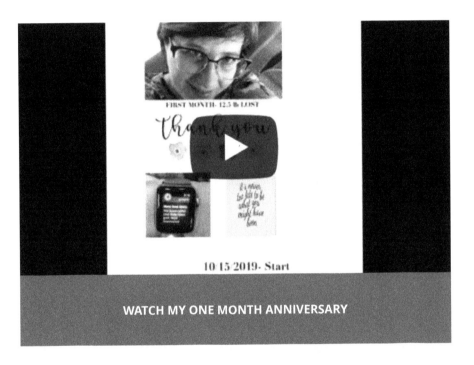

**WATCH MY ONE MONTH ANNIVERSARY**

**https://youtu.be/0n3KZ7MBfYc**

I am so excited.

🩶 I got my new scale and I can see history of my weight loss. My BMI decreased by 1 point in 3 days( since I bought scale).

It's fun to see % of fat, water and muscle mass.

😖 Hope to see my drilling going on 🦵 and soon to feel lighter

🏆 Workout completed before 6 pm.

Love my sour cabbage salad so much 😍

I can eat it for all meals

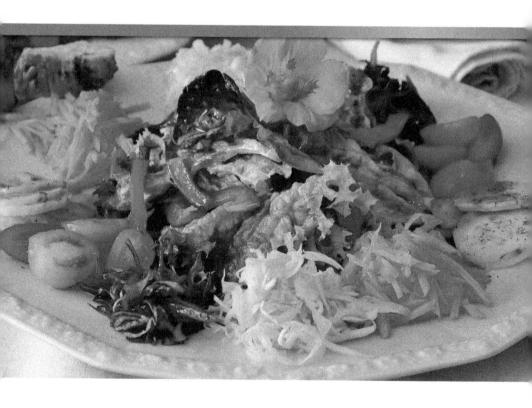

🌚 Happy Tuesday!

No matter what your weight is keep your mind uplifted!😀

🦋 Remember to dream about your dream weight and keep doing everything you can to reach your goal.

I try to do better everyday so I keep closer to my dream.

> **THE BIGGEST ASSET IN THE WORLD IS YOUR MINDSET!**

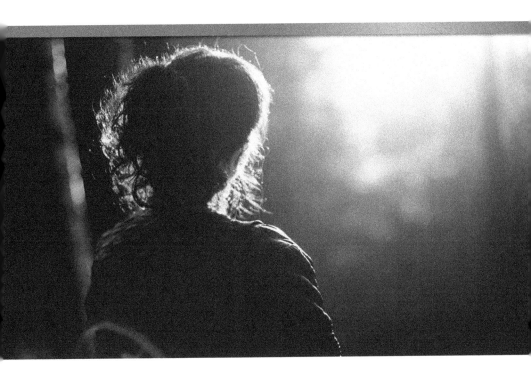

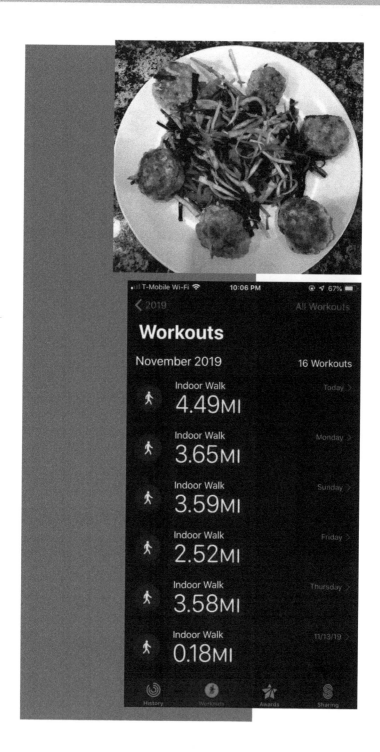

What're your weight loss ideas for Thanksgiving?

- 
- 
- 
- 

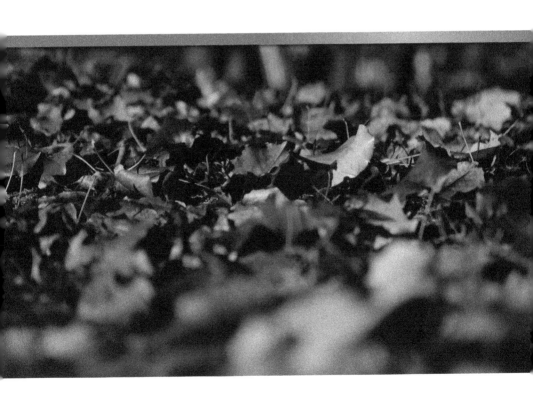

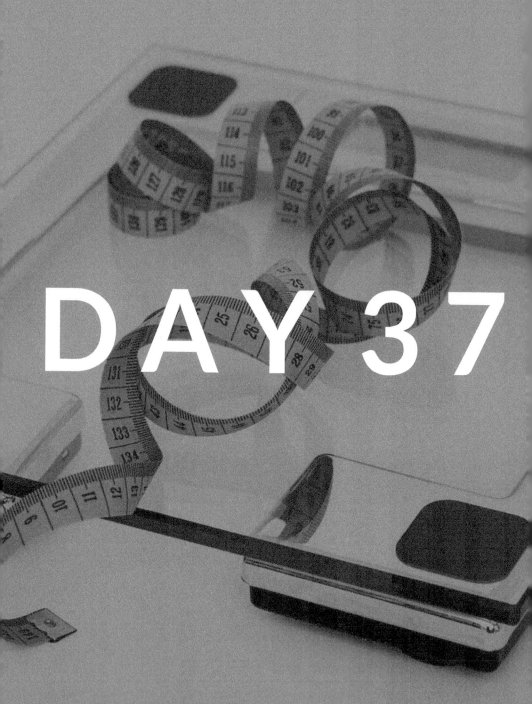

🔑 So, let's pretend that by being in the group and wanted to lose weight sooooo bad you convinced yourself that you are ready.

**This is it**. Today is the perfect day to start.
It doesn't matter if it's Monday or Wednesday.

You are ready! It means you are excited!

> 😯 Where do you start?

*First of all* get an app (lose it, carb counter, ...) or paper journal.

Make sure you have your weight written down.

> What is your goal?
> Why do you want to lose weight?
> Will it change anything in your life if you lose some extra weight?

Imagine yourself at the end of your journey.
Find the best picture of yourself and put it in your journal.

Don't do anything special but *look* at that picture.

This is my first video when I decided today is the day:

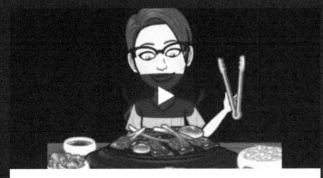

**https://youtu.be/gndCthN8SlY**

**Good morning Saturday!**

Flying 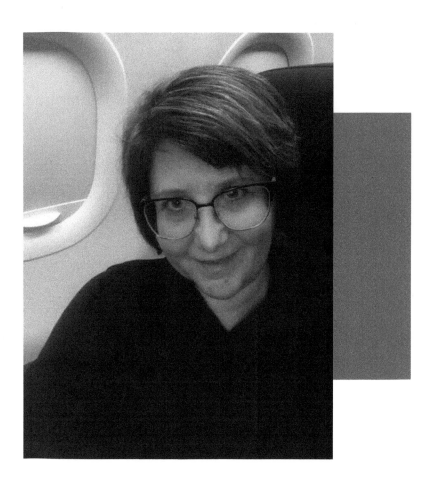 to NY for my cousin's wedding.

Hope to eat portion control in NY.

## I love New York!

Wedding and ceremony was gorgeous!
To be honest, I tried the 🍰 cake and lots of things  from the menu.

I also passed by a bakery with tons of desserts. I didn't buy one cookie.

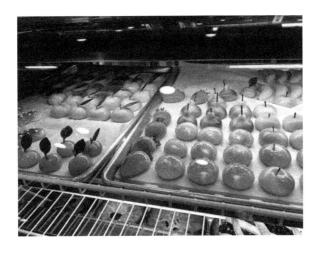

My family had a great table setting and delicious dinner.
I tried...

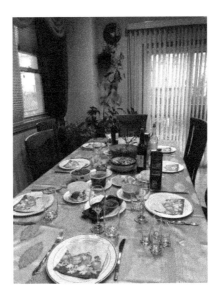

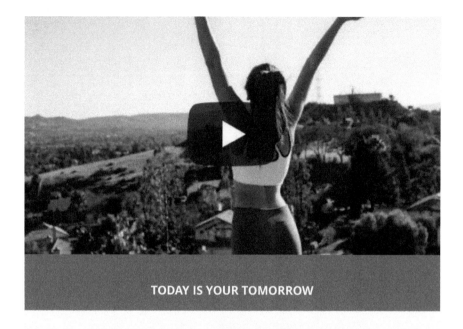

**TODAY IS YOUR TOMORROW**

**https://youtu.be/qSkCQywDipQ**

Homemade Cranberry Sauce #sugarfree

Made with fresh cranberries, wine and stevia

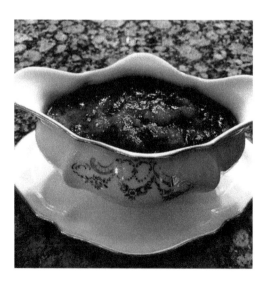

I woke up feeling inspired!

It's amazing to have strong great people around you, people who influence you in a good direction. These people are not doing anything special but they set an example.

🙏I am so grateful for that.

My cousin in NY goes to the gym twice a week at 8 pm. She likes classes.

🏃 Today in the morning I spoke with two of my colleagues. One of them was at the gym at 6 am (Pilates) and another one at 7 am (workouts and weights).

We all know that people lose weight by eating right and exercise alone will not do much. These people are not exercising for weight loss.

Luckily I work 2-8 pm on Tuesday and Thursday. I got back to my routine and did my workout for 1h and 25 min. I felt amazing.

**I am just thankful to have been surrounded by people who are caring about their health and inspire me** 🩶

Sometimes we want to receive positive emotions by giving back to others. I think about that in the same manner as a gift giving. You feel good both ways when you give it or receive it.

If you always receive gifts you should also enjoy giving it.

Positive emotions are so important.

# DAY 42

# DAY 43

Happy Thanksgiving!

Happy Thanksgiving everyone! 🦃🍁🤍

- I am thankful for everything that happens in my life.
- I am grateful for my parents who will bring dishes to my table today.
- I am thankful to my mom in law who never disagrees with me.
- I am thankful for my husband who is my best friend and never says NO.
- I am thankful for my kids.
- I am thankful to my friends who are always there for me.
- I am thankful for my co-workers who are seriously the best people and helping me with lots of stuff.
- I am grateful for my patients who allow me to help them with their health challenges .
- I am also thankful for many of my patients who are athletes, coaches and trainers. I am working out because they inspire me.

🦃🦃🦃🦃🦃🦃🦃🦃🦃🦃

Who is up to a challenge?

Thanksgiving 5K challenge- walk or run 5k on Thanksgiving Day.
Yesterday I walked almost 5 miles for 1 hour and 25 min. It's not easy. Especially on thanksgiving day. But I want it to be my priority so I can do it.

# Happy Thanksgiving!

Happy Thanksgiving everyone!

> 👉 I am thankful for everything that happens in my life.
> 👉 I am grateful for my parents who will bring dishes to my table today.
> 👉 I am thankful to my mom in law who never disagrees with me.
> 👉 I am thankful for my husband who is my best friend
>    and never says NO.
> 👉 I am thankful for my kids.
> 👉 I am thankful to my friends who are always there for me.
> 👉 I am thankful for my co-workers who are seriously the best people
>    and helping me with lots of stuff.
> 👉 I am grateful for my patients who allow me to help them
>    with their health challenges .
> 👉 I am also thankful for many of my patients who are athletes, coaches
>    and trainers. I am working out because they inspire me.

🦃🦃🦃🦃🦃🦃🦃🦃🦃🦃🦃

Who is up to a challenge?

Thanksgiving 5K challenge- walk or run 5k on Thanksgiving Day.

Yesterday I walked almost 5 miles for 1 hour and 25 min. It's not easy. Especially on thanksgiving day. But I want it to be my priority so I can do it.

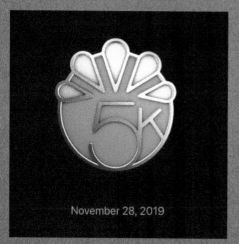

November 28, 2019

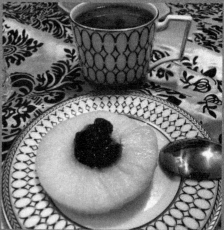

DAY 44

Eating healthy doesn't require a lot of time or too much effort.

I am at my friend's house and love it.

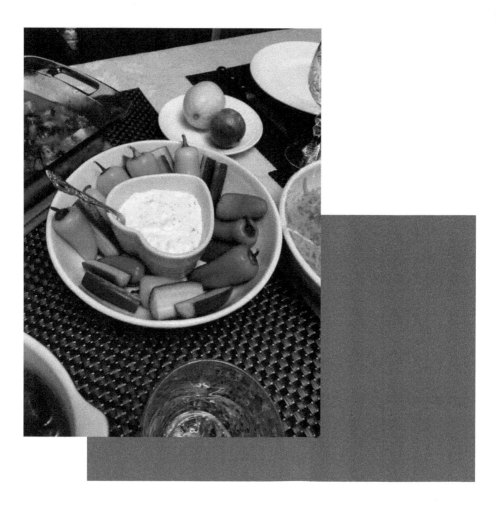

I am lucky other than cardio workouts. Time for structured programs.

I am serious about my weight loss!

It's already December 1st!

This month is one of the toughest months to keep weight down.

But I believe there is nothing impossible!

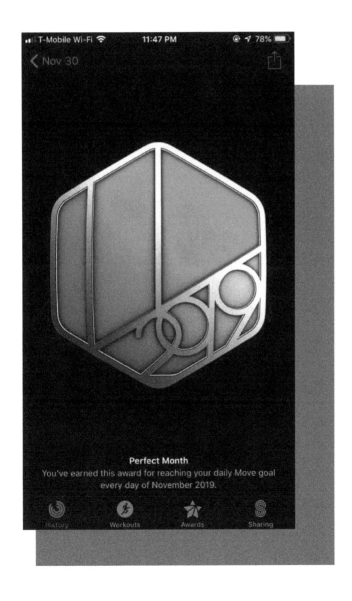

Let's talk about grains. My favorite is buckwheat.

Cholesterol Free
Sugar Free
Good source of Fiber
Low-Fat
Gluten Free
Low Sodium

There is 1g fat, 155 calories, 4.5 g fiber, 5.7 G protein and 34 g carbs in 1 cup of buckwheats

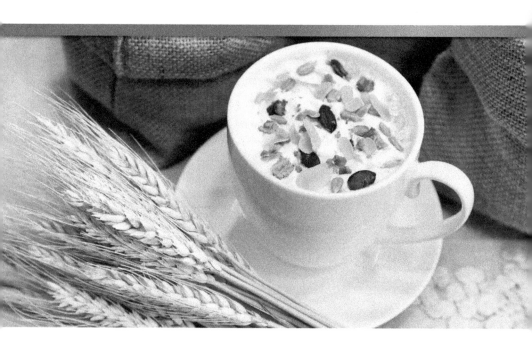

# DAY 48

😍 Power of Positive Thought 😍

I honestly can't believe myself. I completed 50 workouts Since October 15 🏃, . I am almost done watching Biggest loser season 4.

I am addicted to my workouts. Persistence and stepping out of your comfort zone can do it.

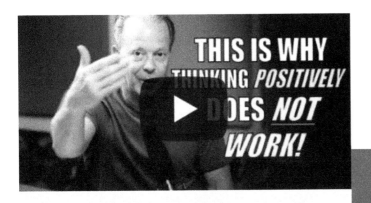

**https://youtu.be/s5Pef_mKQ8s**

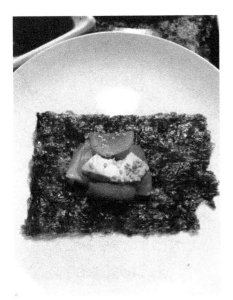

Dinner is served!

Thanks to my husband 🙏

No 🍚 rice for me! Love sashimi

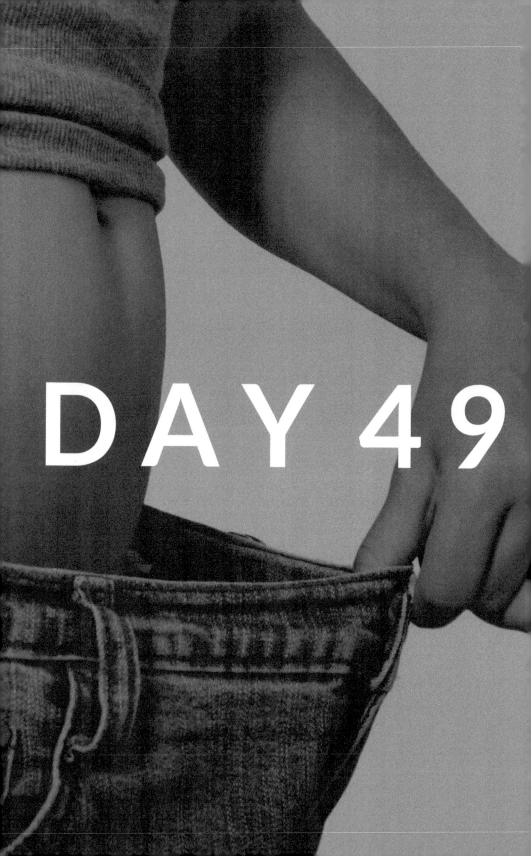

I am excited for upcoming holidays!

27 days until new year!

I better lose those pounds!

🦵 This was my mini workout😂

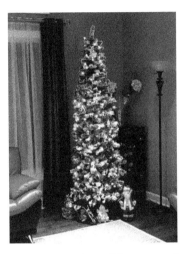

*Let's transmit positive energy!*

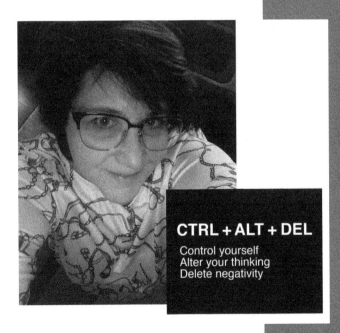

CTRL + ALT + DEL

Control yourself
Alter your thinking
Delete negativity

My fav show will be shown on Tv soon in January again.
The second contestant is from Chicago.
I am excited to watch soon.
Meanwhile working on my weight at home.

It's not easy to lose weight even eating healthy😬
But I will stick to my plan to see results hopefully soon.
Eating cauliflower today.

Who is working out with me?
Finale season 4

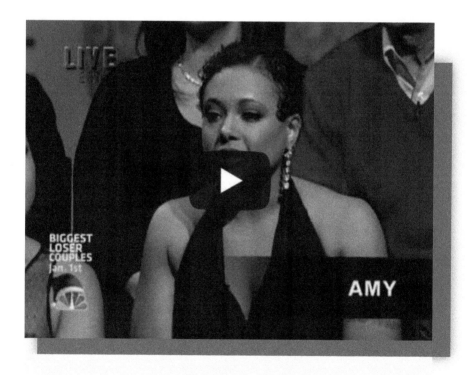

https://youtu.be/-IpyxEPGqMY

You have to do something long enough to see results.
It just takes a long time to lose weight or learn to play music.
I just have to keep trying and be persistent.

What you tell yourself every day will either lift you up or weight you down.

It's a date night. Feed me, honey! 😖
Sushi without rice
No gym today 😂

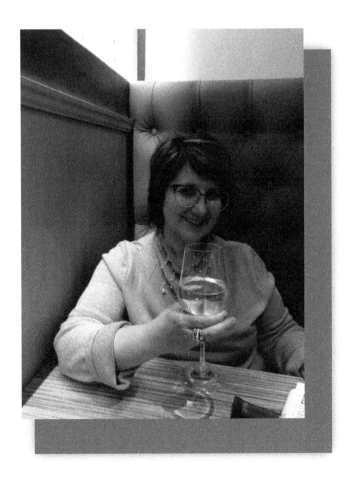

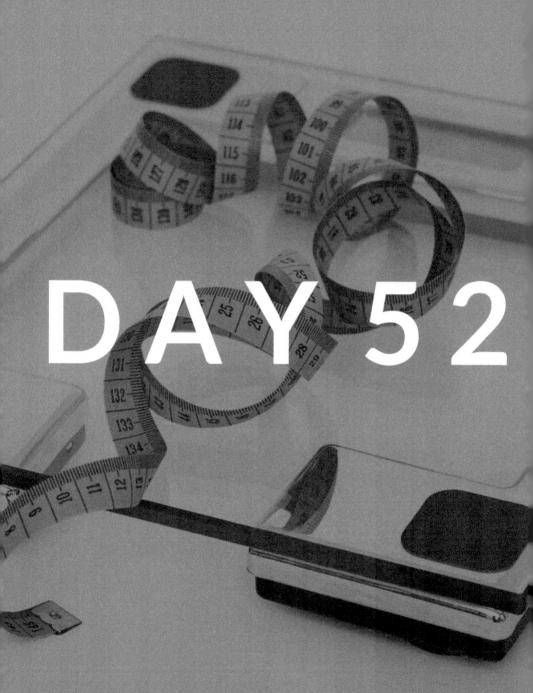

🙏 It's not easy to stay 100% compliant if you have so many friends, events and holidays around.
👉 Just need to remember why I started it, what I want to achieve and what is in front of you:
🩶 Health
👗 Dress

Or maybe something else.

Those 2 are mine.

It's good to believe in being closer to your goat but don't forget to do something about it.

P.S. Sitting at my friend's house surrounded by amazing hosts and delicious food.

Not easy to avoid. Seriously trying.

There are homemade raw vegan cakes.

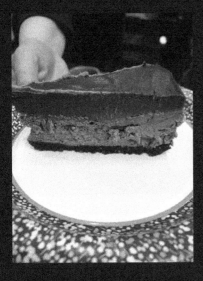

Meet my new friend. I bought a new scale.
Now I will see what's going on in detail.

😬 Does anyone have it?

I love it. It connects to my Apple Health app and shows the history of weight loss, BMI and % of fat, muscle mass, water.

Awesomeness!

# DAY 53

Let's talk about ❄️

Winter

⛩️ According to Chinese Philosophy we should live according to seasons.

❄️ Winter is the most Yin of all seasons. It's the time for more rest, meditate deeply and store physical energy in the form of little added weight. That's why we have tendency to gain more weight or having slower metabolism at this time of the year.

🌊 Water element organs are Bladder and Kidney.

These organs govern water metabolism, adrenal activity and control bladder. They rule sexual organs and reproduction. They provide energy and warmth.
What are the major Kidney imbalances we treat @ our clinic:

☞ all bone problems: #backpain, #kneepain, #spineproblems, #teeth
☞ #hairloss, #premature graying
☞ any #urinary or #reproductive #imbalances
☞ poor #growth, premature #aging
☞ excessive #fear and #insecurity
☞ #hearing loss

What's good to eat during winter? 🍵

🍲 Warm hearty soups made with soup bones and meat, whole grain, roasted nuts, black beans, seaweed, steamed greens. We should cook longer and at lower temperature and with less water.
Salty and bitter flavors bring body heat deeper and lower. Please use salt in moderation still because excess of salt can create coldness and overconsumption of water in the body and thus weaken Winter organs ( Bladder and Kidneys).

Some of the bitter foods include lettuce, turnip, celery, asparagus, oats, quinoa.

Roasted ground chicory is a better substitute for coffee.

Salty foods: miso, seaweed, barley, salt.

# DAY 54

Don't let small minds convince you that your dream is too big.

You can do it.

🖤There is nothing impossible in this world!🖤

I started learning piano 8 weeks ago.

My teacher is so great and I will miss him for 5 month. I had 8 lessons already and even though I am not great yet I want you to hear what I got so far 🎵.

My teacher always reminds me to get rid of tension and enjoy music while playing. It's not easy because I am just a beginner.

⛩️⛩️⛩️⛩️⛩️⛩️

Workout ✅ Happy to watch Biggest Loser season 5.

Lunch: farmer cheese plus feta cheese patties

Dinner: salad with Cajun turkey

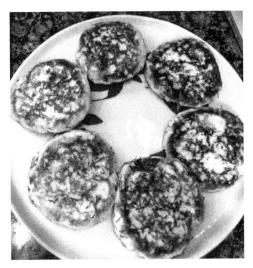 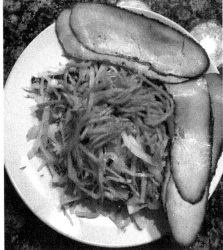

👉 I don't know if you guys have or used this app, but I find it outstanding for daily workouts.

🧘 No equipment needed and you can choose workout for different muscle groups.

It takes 10-20 min for any exercise in the app

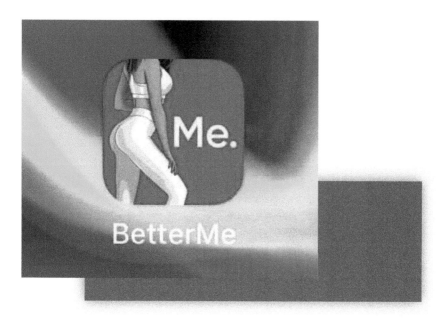

Today I had craving for sandwiches 🥪

So I chose Ezekiel Bread and red caviar. Delish.

I had it for lunch and dinner alone with cabbage salad.

Hope it will not prevent me from losing weight.

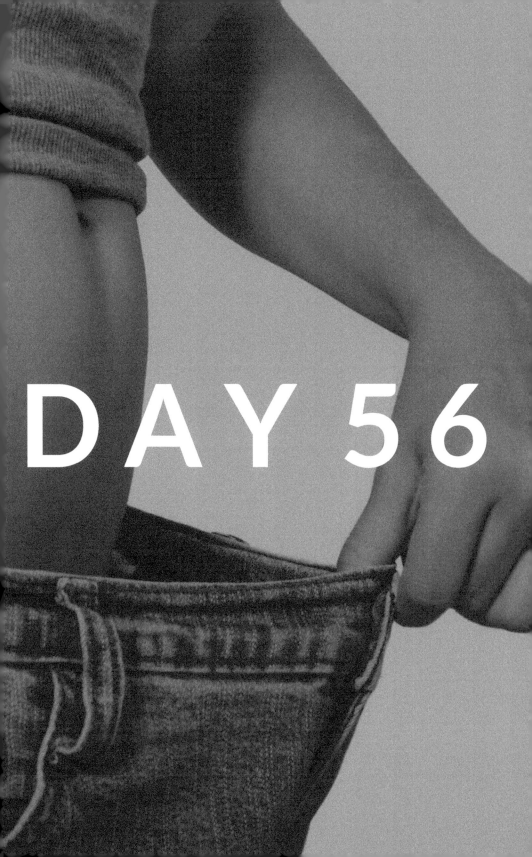

## Why is weight Loss is in your head?

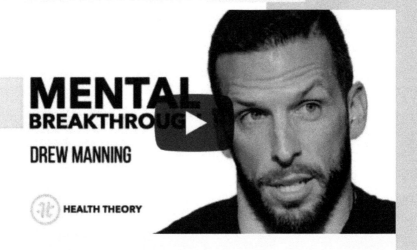

**https://youtu.be/cqwQosiUhTk**

 Simple salad of cauliflower, Cajun chicken, dill and 1 tsp spicy mayo for lunch

Asparagus mushroom soup with 2 meatballs for dinner

Honestly, it's a little bit hard to keep up with portion control.

🙏🙏🙏🙏

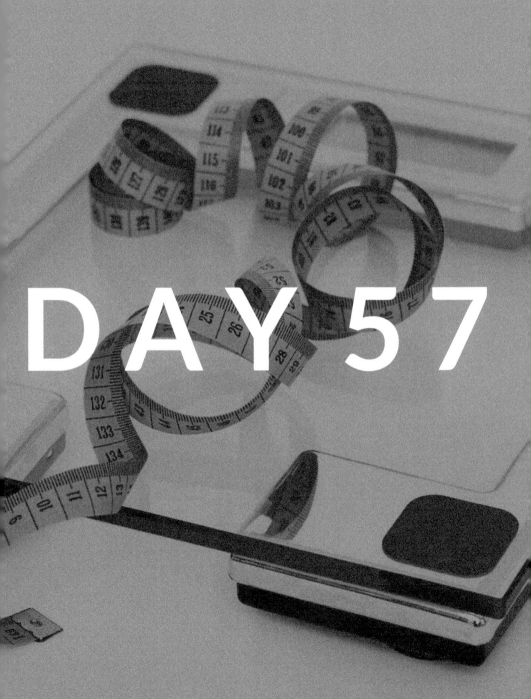

DAY 57

🏃 Getting closer to my weight loss 2 month anniversary! 🤍

Feeling better and lighter 👌

Lunch: salad with white cabbage, celery and carrots. Turkey deli

Dinner: mushroom soup with some of my Asian trout

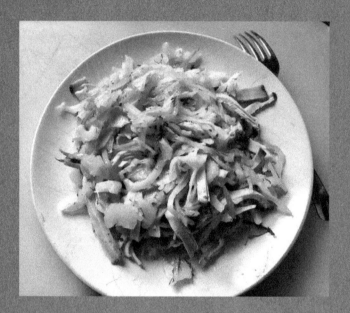

Consistency is more important than perfection.

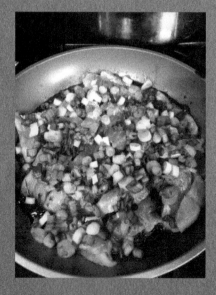 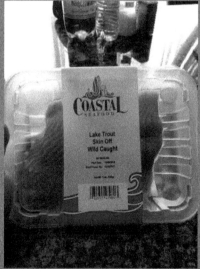

DAY 58

👉Planning for next day is very important

Plan and stick to your available schedule. Commit to a healthy new you!
I made amazing salad: daikon, green apple and cilantro🍏
Fresh and tasty, low in calories.

It takes about 6-8 weeks for the body to adapt to an exercise.

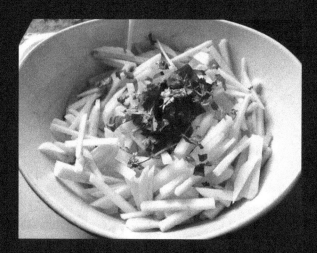

For all of you who survived Friday 13th wishing you have great Saturday 14th😣
If you still struggle just breath in and out. It is what it is.
Let me know if things went crazy today😔
Our office got new shiny look. 🎄

I am so ready for this wonderful holiday season.

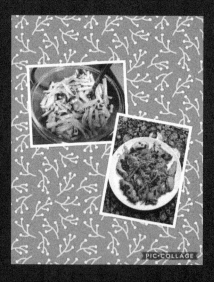

Today is the day to meet with friends and have a good time.

What an awesome bunch of losers!

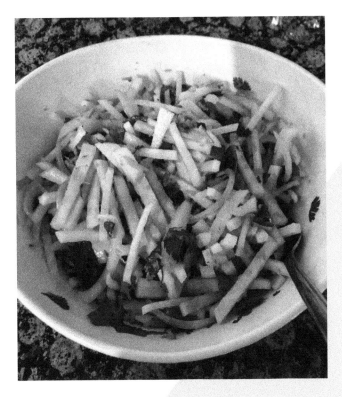

Crash your workout and it will set the tone for the day.

Looking forward to being able to fit into my new clothing. If you can dream it you can do it.

**- Walt Disney**

DAY 59

🍏 Today is my 2 month anniversary of a dedicated weight loss journey!

I am a proud loser of 17.6 lb 💪 🍽️ 🎉

😊 Thank you for being supportive!

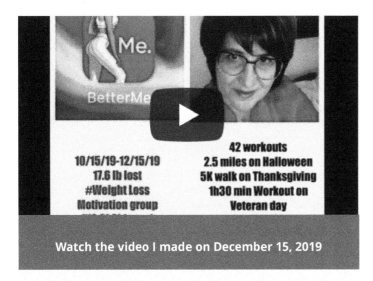

**Watch the video I made on December 15, 2019**

**https://youtu.be/JPFzqnpEG9A**

😵 Did you know that some foods frequently contain mold are coffee, nuts, peanuts, whine and grains?

Mold toxins disrupt the function of insulin and leptin.

Fresh food is important to our health. 🤍

🆔 Let's commit to a healthy 40 days of removing toxins from the body.
It's simple:

- ☑️ 5-10 cups of rainbow 🥕 mostly organic vegetables per day, half raw and half cooked ( we are entering winter season).

- 👌 bitter vegetables with every meal: arugula, radish, dandelion leaves, endive

- 👌 allium vegetables: onion, garlic, leeks

👌 cruciferous vegetables: broccoli, Brussels sprouts, cabbage, cauliflower, kale, radishes

👌 starchy ( 1 serving twice a week) and non starchy vegetables

👌 replace grains with tubers: sweet potatoes, potatoes, yams

☑ Prebiotic fiber: asparagus, Jerusalem artichokes, jicama, onion, leeks, flaxseeds, seaweed

☑ Prebiotic foods: sauerkraut, kefir, kimchi

☑ Spices: turmeric, red pepper and chili, black pepper, ginger, coriander, cardamom, fenugreek, cumin, anise, cinnamon

☑ One 6 Oz serving of berries or cranberry, or grapefruit per day

☑ Protein: 3-4 Oz for women, 6 Oz for men.

Beans, poultry, peas, hemp protein

☑ 2 tbsp per day of healthy fats: coconut oil, olive oil, dark chocolate ( 85%), avocado, olives, wild fish

☑ Fiber: oat bran...Slowly increase to no more than 2-5 g per day. If gas or bloating, back off

☑ Drink: water - half your body weight in oz

Organic herbal tea, green tea, black tea

☑ Intermittent fasting: eating 10 am-6 pm

# DAY 60

Each morning we are born again. What we do today is what matters most.

Buddha

🤍 Love my Monday's- my personal day off

Went for my gym for a treadmill walk- 40 min

2 month ago I started walking with 2.8-3.0 miles per hour.

🚶 🚶 🚶 Today I start with 3.2 m/hr walk

Every 5 min I increased to 1 more mile and went up to 3.7m/hr which is very fast for me. I tried not to think or look at the clock and concentrate on my best show- Biggest loser season 5( 3).

🙏 People were punished for touching treadmill handles so hands would remain free for harder workouts. Once they touch everyone in the room should run 5 more min.

After 3.7 speed I pushed back every 5 min. 3.5 felt like a very amazing brisk walk and 3.4 like I am on a fashion podium💃

I watched a comedy movie yesterday about a "fat" girl who wanted to run a marathon. So anything is possible if you believe.

Brittany Runs a Marathon

Honestly, I like my workouts.

🏋️ Seriously, once you start moving and have at least a little bit of competitive drive to compete with yourself we can do anything we want to accomplish. Even if you have time on Saturday and Sunday do it. It only takes 30 min. You will feel better.


👉 Breakfast: coffee
👉 Lunch: daikon and green apple 🍏 salad
👉 Dinner, date night: riceless sushi

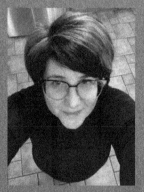
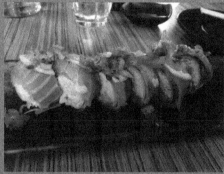

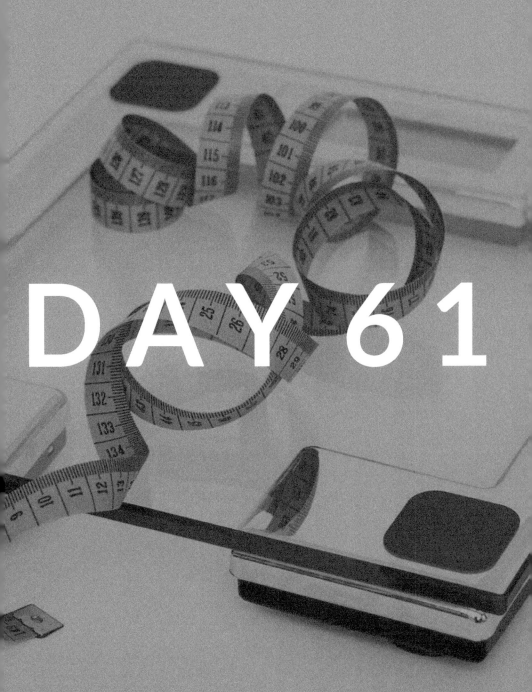

DAY 61

Train your mind to see the good in everything. Positivity is a choice. The happiness of your life depends on the quality of your thoughts.

🌱 Very green fresh salad: cucumbers, daikon, avocado, green apple, cilantro, lemon, feta, olive oil, almonds

Branzino fish is sooo good. Hard to stop. But I am good. I just had 2 pieces.

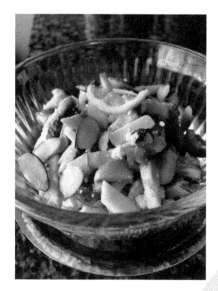
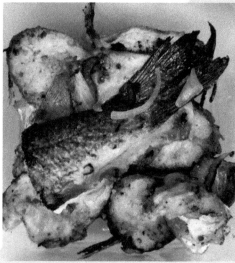

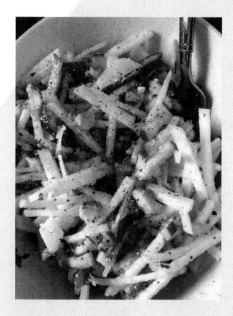

# DAY 62

🖤Today I am very thankful for my patient's advice to download this app. It helps to change any workout to a more productive exercise.

You don't have to be a runner to use it. As a matter of fact I never run in my entire life. It connects with the iPhone, guides you and gives you feedback. Not free but cool 😎 fun thing to use.

🥚Yesterday I made a new recipe in my Pressure cooker. Egg bites resemble delicious Starbucks egg bites. I had one with salad for lunch.

🍴Dinner: Salad and another egg bite.

Snack: needed some protein so got my fish recipe ready to roll in my mouth.

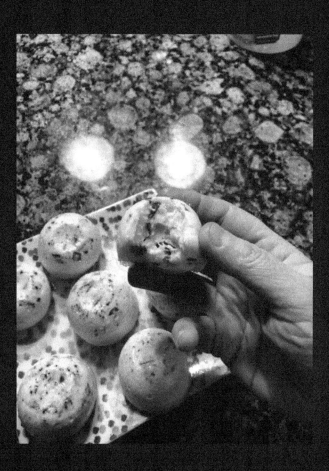

The best thing I ever did is to believe in myself 2 month ago.

A year from now you will wish you had started today.

💰 💸 💵 Another way to lose weight if nothing works...

Pay yourself or join HealthyWage to receive money for losing weight.

I am thinking about it.

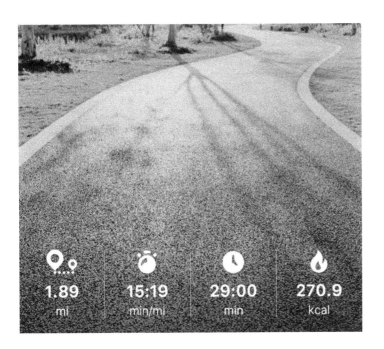

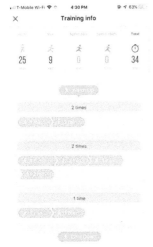

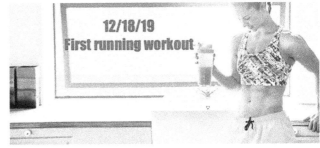

🎄 Intermittent running 🏃, is fun.

I am planning to lose weight during this holiday season.

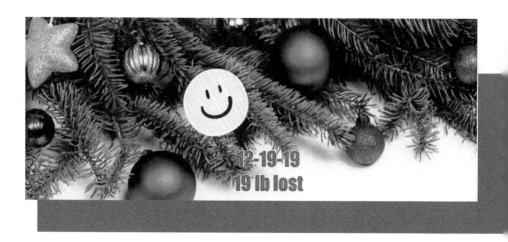

Great advice: don't stress and have fun

It takes 6 weeks to get used to some new activity or change in schedule.

I am definitely on the 2nd day of running workout before my work.

Today is a new day. It's OK if you failed yesterday.

Ways to stay motivated in December:

Workout to holiday music

Happy Friday!!!

🍷 All I want for this Holiday Season is Metabolismo Accelerato!

🥕 Snacking is important. Especially around 10 pm😴

I like nuts or apples. What's your favorite snack?

100 calories are only 25 pistachios, 14 almonds, 11 cashews.

😍 Happy Friday everyone and Shabbat Shalom to all who celebrate.

🤔 Have to remember to be mindful during weekends and holidays.

💪 It's important to remind yourself why you are trying to lose weight. Sometimes weight goes back a few lb for no reason. Stop and evaluate. You know Why!😂

As long as we are in progress! 🍷🙏

Sometimes you think you are not improving. Check an old picture of you and see how far you have come.

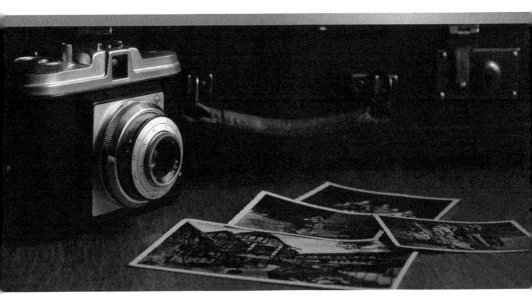

DAY 65

♡ ♡ ♡ ♡ ♡ Happy Saturday!
😬 Getting ready for a busy day of work!

Plan and commit!
I always prepare my lunch and dinner the day before. If I don't it could go unexpected.
My plan is to use my Gym 4 days a week.
Monday, Tuesday, Wednesday and Thursday.

I am glad I went for a walk yesterday on Friday!
Felt amazing!

It's easy to say that you want to lose weight. Eat better and workout more.
But unless You  plan and commit, it will just stay a dream.

♡ I am so thankful for our patients and friends who brought and sent Flowers and these wonderful and Yummy things.

😬 Sharing is caring so I left some in the office and gave my receptionist some and got myself something. My family will love it.

🍷 it's Saturday eve and we are going out.
Time spent in a good company is very precious.
I am going to have my fav salad at Kamehachi in Northbrook.
🏃 No gym today.

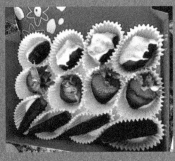

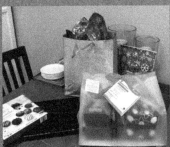

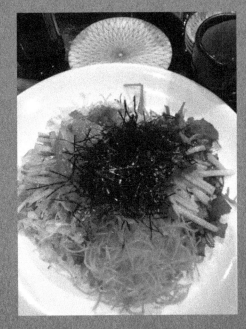

Some people rent on Sunday. I don't.

How about the Chanukah Challenge?

8 days of daily workouts?

I am in!

1st one

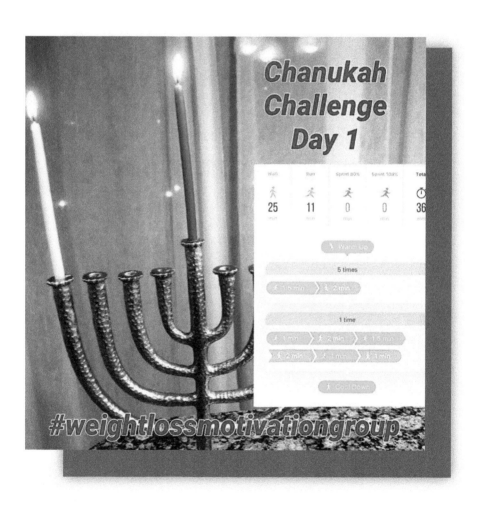

Hanukkah 8 days 🕎 Challenge

@weight_loss_group_ns_suburbs

Day 2

🤤 No more latkes for me!

🍯🥔🥗🥩🍩

You don't have to go fast, you just need to go!

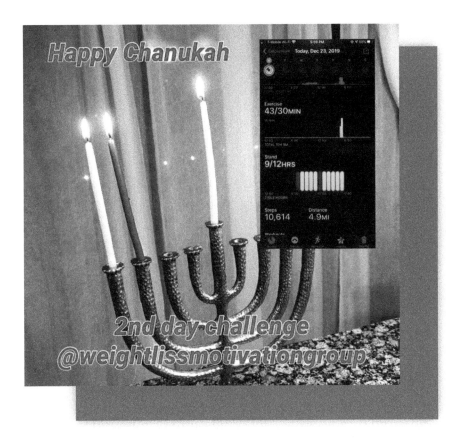

🎄 Good morning!

When it comes to a holiday season it becomes more difficult to maintain weight, not to lose it.

🐟 Eating more fish for protein makes it easier. Here is my branzino creation. It's delicious.
🍷 My cousin invited us for the second day of Chanukah and cooked a very healthy dinner.

For dessert I had half of dark chocolate candy and coffee.

Merry Christmas to everyone and Happy Hanukkah!

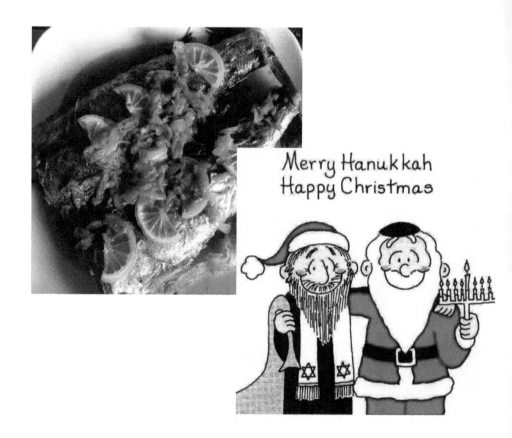

Merry Hanukkah
Happy Christmas

# DAY 69

Merry Christmas and Happy Hanukkah to all of you!!!!🎁

Wishing everyone great health and awesome happy Attitude for everything we do! 🤍

I celebrate my 26 Anniversary today! Only some people could marry on Christmas when everything is closed.

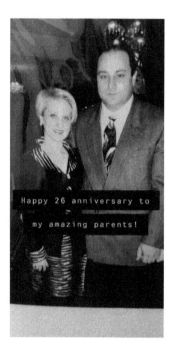

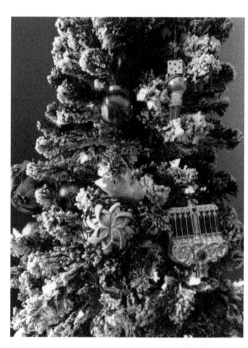

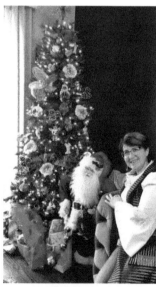

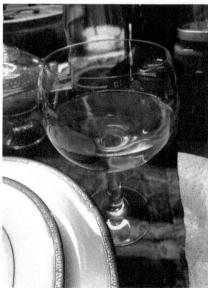

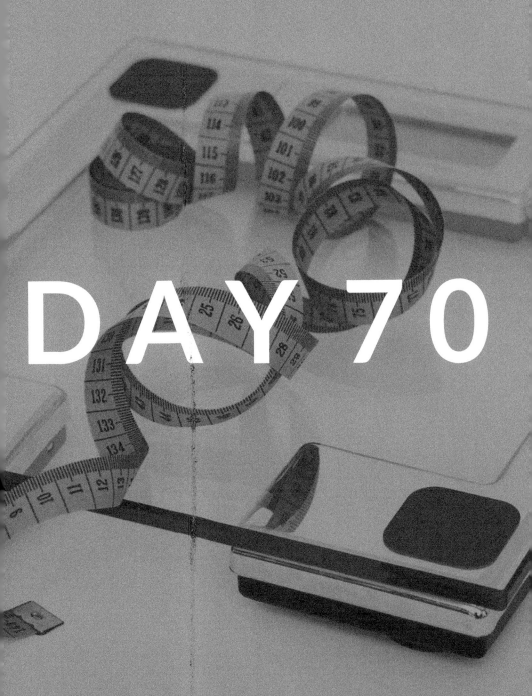

DAY 70

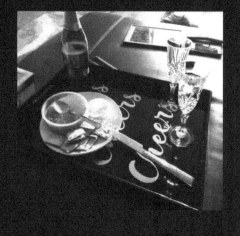

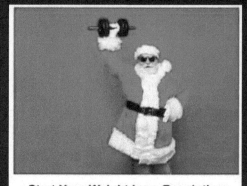

😄Not eating dessert is not a problem!🍫
It's tough to lose weight during holidays!
I am still trying...🚶
Calling my friend to go for a walk together! Hope you are eating healthy and exercising

DAY 71

I am going to complete my workout before my workday!

If you need to boost energy, blend together 1 carrot, 1 apple, 3 slices of ginger and 1 teaspoon of turmeric.

Done with my workout. Better late than never. I thought I could do it before work but ☕ coffee won.

Very proud of myself for exercising before going out with my family and friends. Now it's easier to make healthy choice. 🔪🥒🍎🍷

Hope you guys have a good time.

Happy Friday !

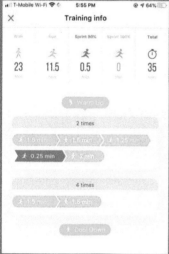

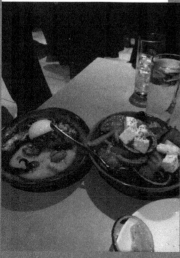

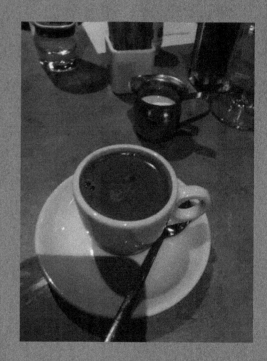

🖤Today is my son's 17th birthday!

Mama needs to feel young and energetic after work !🤪

After all if we are not healthy how can we take care of our kids😄

Healthy food + moving = happy feeling 😄

I bought my son favorite dessert: whole food raspberry chocolate mini tart🧁

I workout on my treadmill so I can smell that🍫

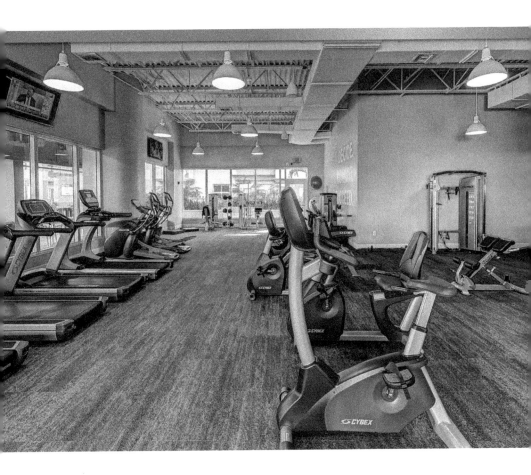

A goal without a plan is just a wish.

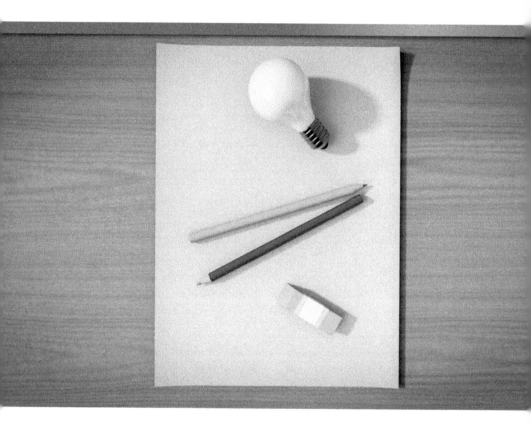

Great salad made of beets, carrots, almonds and prunes
Food is the most abused anxiety drug.
Exercise is the most underutilized antidepressant.

- From Tips on Getting Fit and Healthy

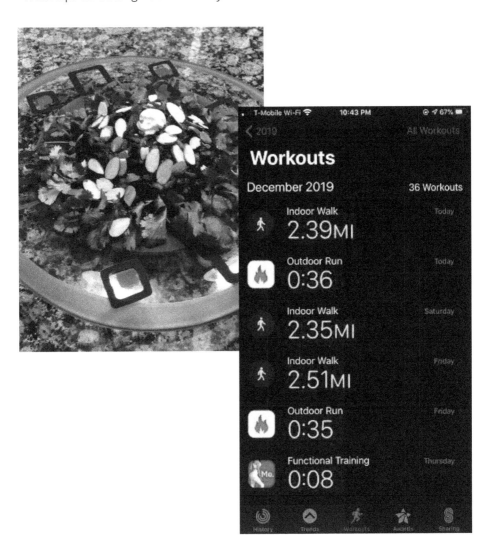

🎉Happy New Year!!!🎉🌲

🌍Almost Everything can be healthy in moderation!

Even a glass of champagne or two for New Year!

Enjoy your company and thank you for supporting me and each other in 2019!🙏

See you in 2020! Wishing you health and happiness!

Wishing you all happy and healthy New Year!

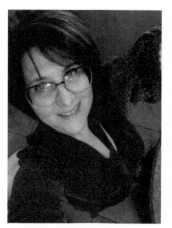
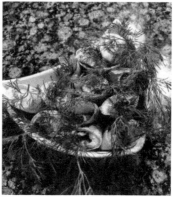

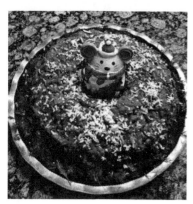

Happy 2020!!!!! 🍰
Believe in Miracles!
I lost 2 lb after New Year Celebration!!!! 🤍 🙌 🎈 🍾 🍷 🎁 😂 🎄 😄 ☕

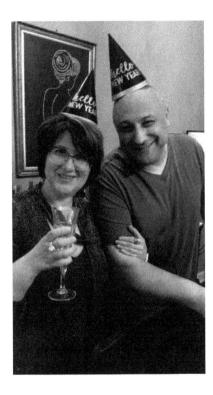

I am proud of my New Workout in 2020! ✅
I picked up everything on the floor piece by piece , one by one! 🏋️
Not easy but worth it! 🤣
Clean eating today
B. Coffee

L. Cauliflower wrap with salmon
Snack. Mandarin
D. Branzino fish

Let's make a difference in 2020!

Who is with me?

2020 will bring 365 opportunities to all of you! 365 opportunities!

👉 Love my detox salad: daikon, green apple 🍏, carrots 🥕, cilantro and olive oil

🏃 Walked on treadmill for 40 min

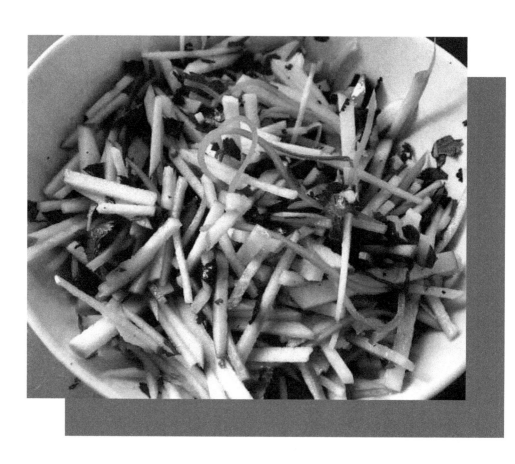

Happy Friday, everyone!

Today is the day to eat less and move more!

I have new January challenges - 22 workouts in January and accomplish 3 goals: move, exercise and stand for 7 consecutive days

Best competition is with yourself

Friday night!
Wine and painting!
Very calming!

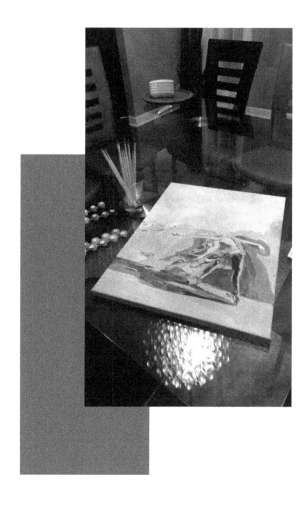

I can not wait for our office holiday 🎄 party today🎉

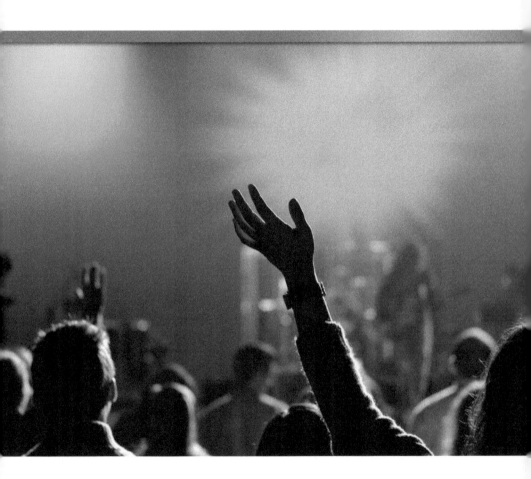

# DAY 80

It has been a difficult time for me being surrounded by festive food choices. Trying my best!

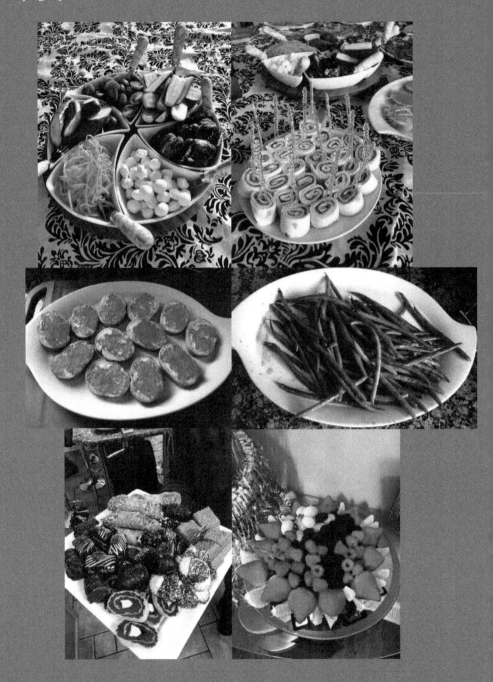

I woke up with excruciating pain in my leg.

I needled myself and decided to walk on the treadmill after.

40 min of brisk walking is absolutely fantastic.

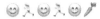

Eating clean and healthy!

Holidays are O V E R !

Just clean clean clean eating!

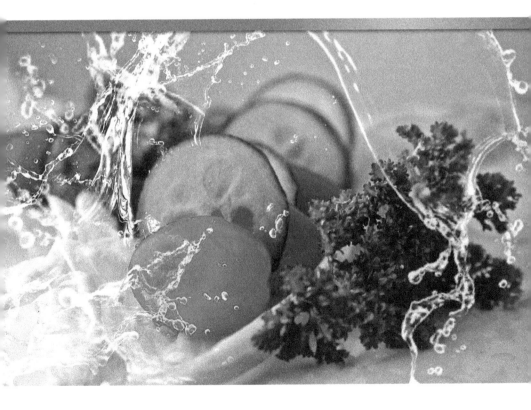

I woke up with excruciating pain in my leg.
I needled myself and decided to walk on the treadmill after.
40 min of brisk walking is absolutely fantastic.
😊 🏃 😊 🏃 😊 🏋
Eating clean and healthy!


Holidays are O V E R !
Just clean clean clean eating!

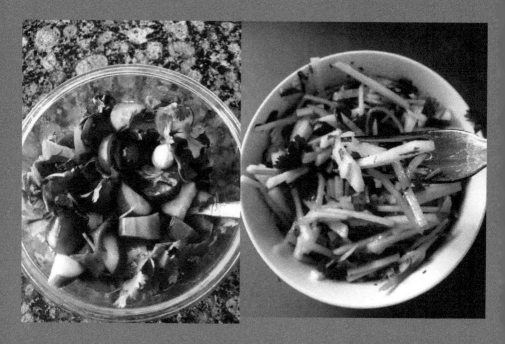

Surround yourself with people who pushed you to do and be better!

DAY 82

Merry Orthodox Christmas to all of my friends who celebrate this holiday. Wishing you many blessings for health, joy and prosperity!

Portion control again

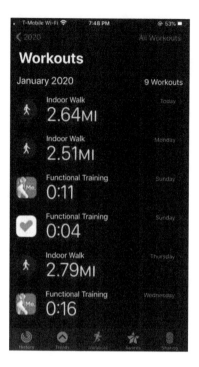

What was on your plate today?

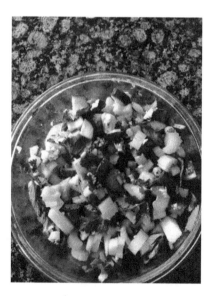

☝Be consistent in everything you want to achieve!
Do it long enough to experience the desired effect!
Who is with me today?

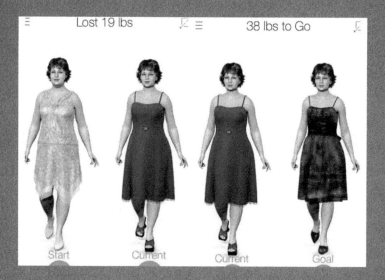

| Lost 19 lbs | | 38 lbs to Go | |
| --- | --- | --- | --- |
| Start | Current | Current | Goal |

Omg!
🙏🙏🙏🙏 Today something happened to me
I had awesome lunch 👇
But then right before dinner 3-4 pm I had: cheese, raspberry, meatballs, coffee, cheese, raspberries.....
God help me!!!
I hope you are stronger than me✊
Please eat right ☝

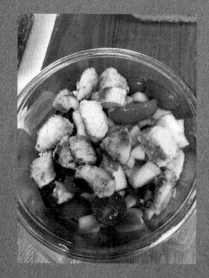

# DAY 84

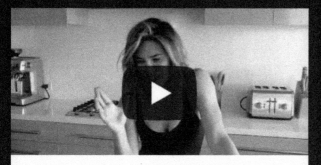

**https://youtu.be/R5_TDnffZvA**

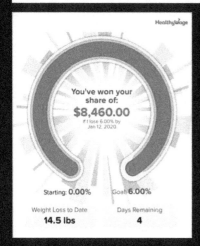

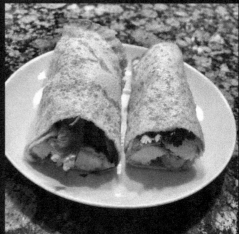

I was a competitive player for HealthWedge and I won a share. I can only imagine that it could be about $60 or $50. I am really proud of it.

Amazingly enough I lost 1 lb since yesterday.😛
🍗 Made myself amazing lunch- chicken wrap
Egg cauliflower wrap ( Costco 30 cal) with tbsp of hummus (80 cal) and leftover chicken breast (80 cal)
😋 Looks great and tasty! All I need

🍷 Celebrating with my family my 🏋 20 lb 🏋 loss

🤭 Except I eat salad with raw fish.

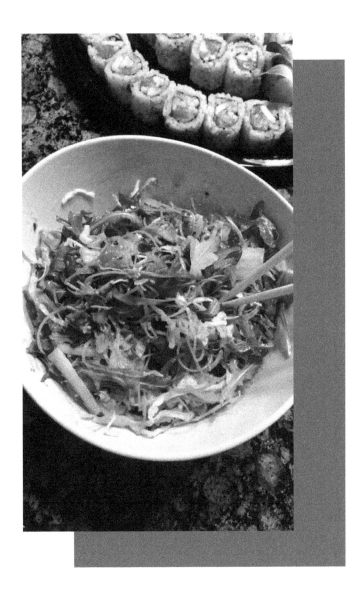

# DAY 86

Happy Saturday!
Love my busy schedule!🤣
It's so easy to stay away from food!
😍Happily I got invited to my friend so I must be careful!

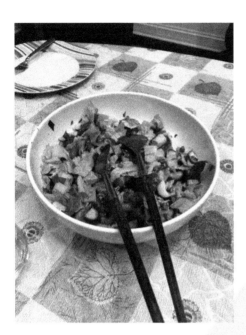
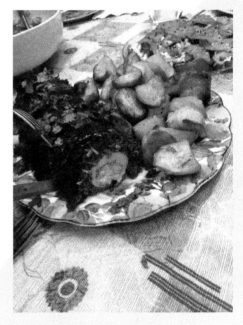

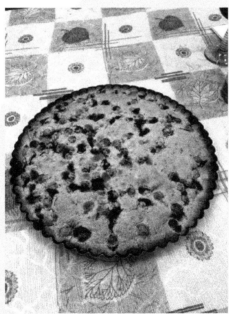

Good morning and Happy Sunday!!! 🖤 We got ⚪!

I am extremely happy to wake up and see that I didn't gain any weight yesterday. It's absolutely awesome to go out or be with friends partying anywhere on Fridays, Saturdays and Sundays.
Since October 15, 2019 I learn a few things:

   ☞ Eat healthy food
   ☞ Know your portion
   ☞ Move more
   ☞ There is no secret in weight loss or magic 💊
   ☞ I can lose weight on major holidays:

Halloween 👻 (no dessert challenge ☑)
Thanksgiving 🍗 ( lost 1 lb ☑ )
Rosh Hashana 🎉
Yom Kippur 🐺
Veterans Day 🙏 ( 5K ☑ )
8 days of Hanukkah( toughest time- lost 1 lb ☑ )
Christmas 🎄

Holiday parties 🎁
Birthdays 🍷
New Year ( list 2 lb ☑ )

   ☞ I can lose weight when I go out 🍷
   ☞ Every day is a new opportunity ✌
   ☞ Love yourself 😊
   ☞ Don't feel sorry for yourself
   ☞ Surround yourself with people who are positive
     and supportive I am 💐.
   ☞ Try to encourage other people. We all need support
   ☞ Celebrate your success. I do it every time 🎉🎁
   ☞ Enjoy your life

DAY 88

♡ Bought new plates and cups for me and my family! 2020 with new plates and cups.
Love to get rid of old and new!

😊 Made delicious farmer cheese cake today:

Mixed 16 Oz farmer cheese, 3 eggs, monk fruit sweetener, 1 tsp of baked powder and 3/4 cup of flax milk. Pour into a form and top with fresh thin sliced apples. Baked at 390 F for 40 min

Delicious

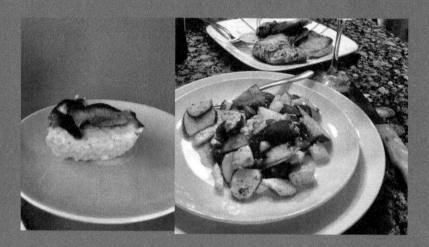

♡ Today me and my family will have homemade winter soup 🥘 Borsch: beef broth, 3 bay leaves, 🥕, 🧅, beets, cabbage, 🥔,white beans.
Serve with a spoon of sour cream.
😄 Patience and love is needed to make this soup.
Filling and healthy: complex meal: protein, carbs, fat and fiber.

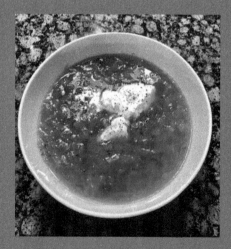

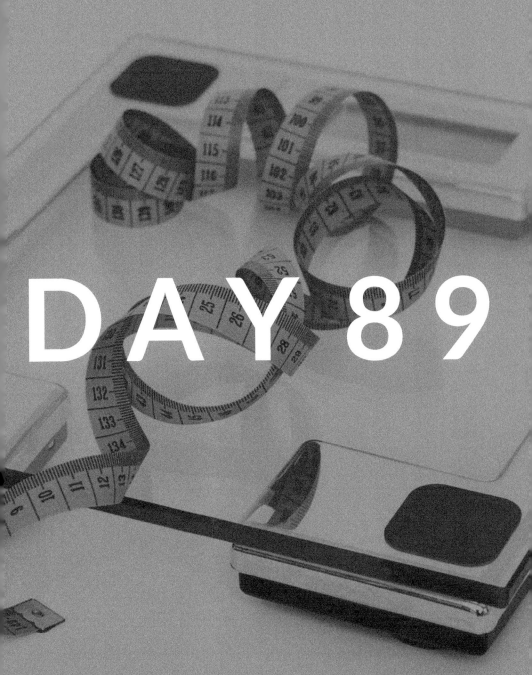

DAY 89

Today's prayer..... God please let me look like #JLo when I'm 50. Amen 🙏

Eating soup twice a day😄

Creating Calorie deficit is important.

Calories in, calories out!

Tomorrow my 3 month Anniversary!😍😍😍

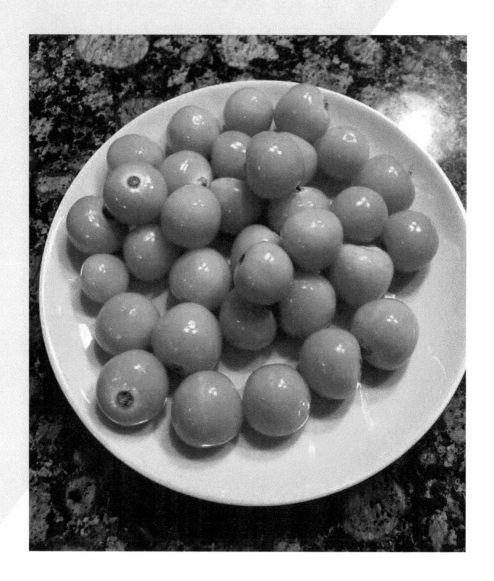

DAY 90

Today is my 3rd month Weight Loss Anniversary

**Please watch my video**

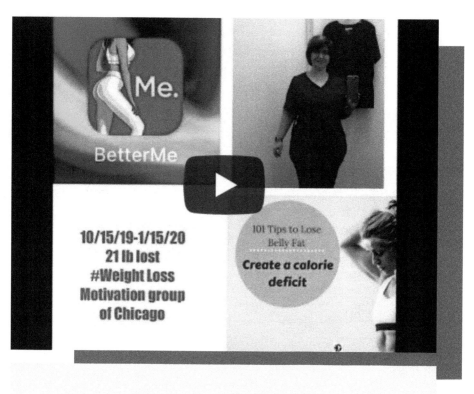

https://youtu.be/tjSRNhR7XOw

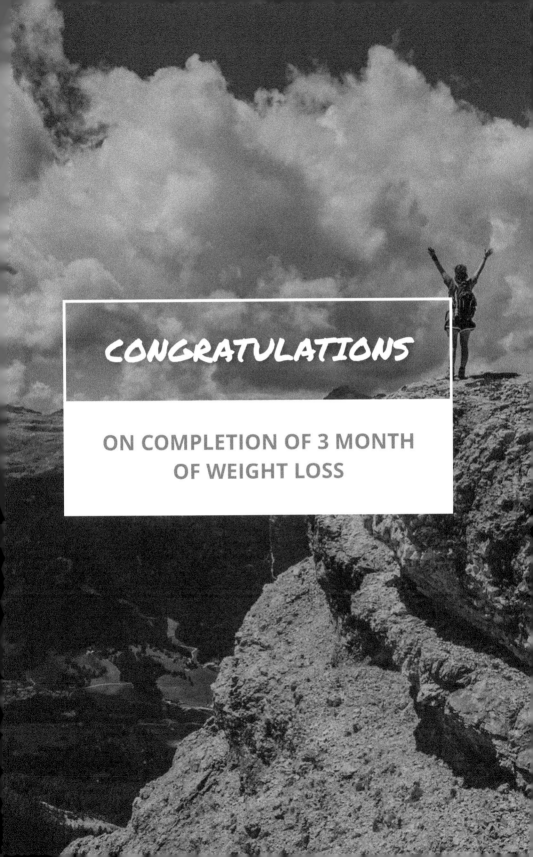

# CONGRATULATIONS

## ON COMPLETION OF 3 MONTH OF WEIGHT LOSS

CPSIA information can be obtained
at www.ICGtesting.com
Printed in the USA
JSHW040522180920
7994JS00004B/52